D1759101

This family tr.... .....
the parish registers of the parish of St Mary,
Chester, and from census returns for 1841–1881.

*No prefix to date indicates date of christening*

Prefixes to dates
m = married
f = funeral
b = buried
† = illegitimate
Ro = registry office
n = family notation

[ ]   Detailed in Chapter 1, Fig 3.

\*     Ellen had 3 illegitimate children. Peter's father is
      merely recorded as "Fisherman"

Holy Trinity

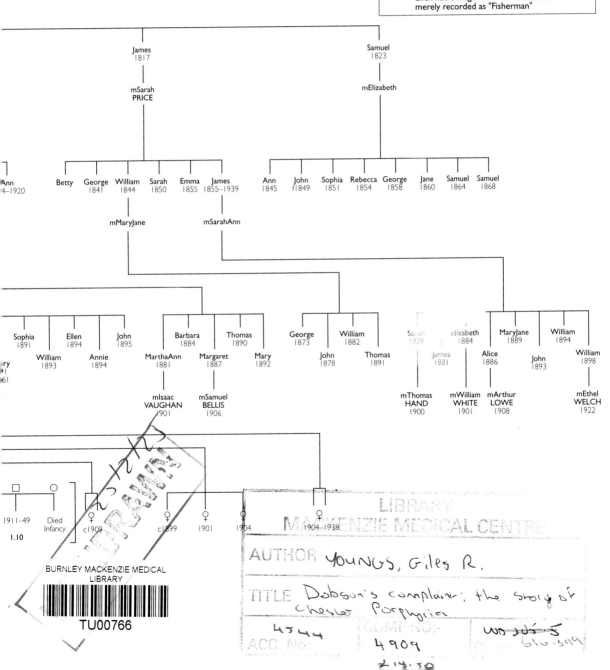

# Dobson's complaint

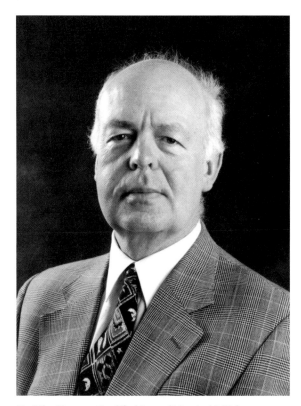

Dr Giles Youngs. Qualified in medicine in 1966 from
Gonville and Caius College, Cambridge, and the London
Hospital. He was introduced to gastroenterology by Ian
Bouchier and Sheila Sherlock at the Royal Free Hospital and
completed his training with Duncan Colin-Jones and John
Bamforth at Southampton. He was appointed Consultant
Physician and Gastroenterologist to the Chester Hospitals in
1974. He has served as Royal College of Physicians
Regional Adviser (Mersey) and on the College Council.

# Dobson's complaint

The story of the Chester Porphyria

*Edited by*

**Giles R Youngs**

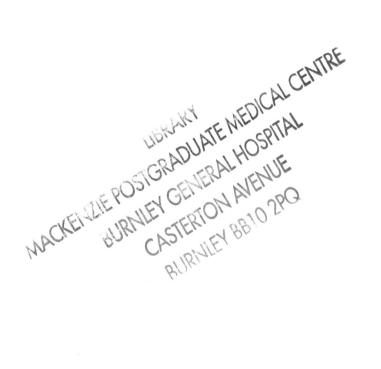
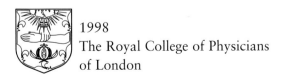
1998
The Royal College of Physicians
of London

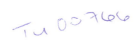

## Cover illustrations

The picture on the front cover is taken from a postcard of a 19th century print, showing salmon fishermen with their nets by the River Dee, Chester.

The engraving, "Graves", shown on the back cover is by Aishlyn Tracy Youngs. It conveys the sadness experienced by the Dobson family, many members of which died at a premature age.

## Endpapers

The Dobson family tree. (Researched by Andrew McDonagh.)

**Royal College of Physicians of London**
**11 St Andrews Place, London NW1 4LE**

**Registered Charity No. 210508**

Copyright © 1998 Royal College of Physicians of London

ISBN 1 86016 047 6

Designed by Merriton Sharp, London

Printed in Great Britain by The Lavenham Press Ltd, Lavenham, Sudbury, Suffolk

# What others have said

*The Chester kindred's acute hepatic porphyria is inherited, Porphyrion's liver lesion was acquired; both can prove fatal*

Then Porphyrion leaped into Heaven from the great pyramid of rocks which the giants had piled up, and none of the Gods stood his ground. Only Athene adopted a posture of defence. Rushing by her, Porphyrion made for Hera, whom he tried to strangle; but, wounded in the liver by a timely arrow from Eros's bow, he turned from anger to lust, and ripped off Hera's glorious robe. Zeus, seeing his wife was about to be outraged, ran forward in jealous wrath, and felled Porphyrion with a thunderbolt. Up he sprang, but Heracles, returning to Phelgra in the nick of time, mortally wounded him with an arrow.

Robert Graves: The Giants' Revolt, The Greek Myths, 1992

*Porphyria misdiagnosed*

When somebody dies from hysteria in this province she usually suffers from acute porphyria.
(*Waldenström quoting a colleague from Swedish Lapland*)

J Waldenström: The porphyrias as inborn errors of metabolism, 1957

*Porphyrics spurned*

The vicious acerbity of the conduct of porphyrinuric termagants makes it difficult at times to treat them on a medical ward. Nurses dislike caring for them. They are a troublesome group of patients and kindle feelings of hatred and aggression in the most urbane physicians.

RM Kark: Clinical aspects of the major porphyrinopathies, 1957

# Preface

I was fortunate to be appointed consultant physician and gastro-enterologist to the Chester hospitals in 1974. The subsequent burden and heat of the day have been tempered by my interest in the Chester porphyria kindred. The fascination of family members' medical and social histories has caused this interest to expand, just as the kindred itself continues to expand – from a marriage in 1888 to over 300 scions now. The spark that ignited my researches was the accusation by a family member that I was as ignorant of porphyria as all the other local hospital and general medical practitioners. The fuel was the growing realisation that not only had this inherited condition caused devastating morbidity and mortality to a large but close-knit Chester kindred, but also that the victims had presented with their symptoms to a wide variety of hospital specialists and general practitioners at many different venues in the city. The result was that the family, who had suffered the death of several young members, were all too aware of their collective plight, but their medical advisers were both unaware of the size of the problem and also unversed in the diagnosis of the condition which notoriously, with hindsight, mimics more common and less serious maladies. The family members therefore received inaccurate or delayed diagnoses, incorrect death certificates, unsympathetic consultations, and accusations of hysteria. An added bonus to my quest was that, with the help of colleagues in Glasgow, we subsequently showed that the genetics and biochemistry of the Chester porphyria are apparently unique.

It is ironic that porphyria has become my hobby within medicine because I remember having to swot up its biochemical complexities the night before each MRCP examination. My knowledge was ephemeral, but fortunately generations of medical registrars (co-authors of this monograph) quickly realised that I am a macro-gastroenterologist. I find it difficult to grasp the intricacies of any particle much smaller than a gallstone, and am happier wielding a gastroscope than a restriction enzyme. I am grateful for their help and enthusiasm.

This book attempts to convey to the reader some of the fascination and pathos of the kindred's story, rather than act as an exhaustive reference work on porphyria. Robert Browning's lines capture a flavour of the agonies experienced by the family and of the ardour which drove me to describe them, often in the middle of the night – for I have become Porphyria's lover!

> The rain set early in to-night,
>     The sullen wind was soon awake,
> It tore the elm-tops down for spite,
>     And did its worst to vex the lake:
>     I listen'd with heart fit to break.
> When glided in Porphyria;...
>
> Porphyria's love: she guessed not how
>     Her darling one wish would be heard.
> And thus we sit together now,
>     And all night long we have not stirred,...

(From *Porphyria's Lover* by Robert Browning)

GILES YOUNGS
*May 1998*

# Foreword

Few encounters can be so stimulating – or so salutary – for the physician as meeting a 'client' who not only suggests, correctly, the probable diagnosis of his or her own malady but, incidentally, conveys the expert consultant's ignorance thereof, and adds to his discomfiture by rejecting his well meant but inappropriate reassurance as to the likelihood of a favourable outcome. This is precisely what occurred in 1980 in the outpatient department of Chester Royal Infirmary. It became apparent that the unfortunate patient was in all probability suffering from a form of acute intermittent porphyria, the elucidation of which presented a great challenge. As anticipated, each of her subsequent readmissions posed difficult management problems. Her immediate family history confirmed the gravity of this inherited disease, with father and brother already 'untimely dead'. The kindred were well aware of the import of 'Dobson's complaint' – an eponym conveyed by a family doctor to Giles Youngs and his team.

An intriguing aspect proved to be the recognition that in Chester the families principally affected came from the almost closed community of Dee salmon fishermen – not famous respecters and upholders of the law. How much of their antisocial behaviour could be attributed to the hardships of their precarious calling and how much to the insidious effects of this disease, whose unexpectedly high incidence is consistent with an initially incestuous union?

The study of death certificates, parish records and similar sources (perhaps made easier by the fact that the fisher families tended not to migrate), and even accepting incomplete or frankly erroneous diagnoses, provided pointers to the morbidity of the complaint. More recent work has uncovered the high incidence of life-threatening renal, hypertensive, cardiovascular and cerebrovascular disease. Zorka Bekerus' initial experience, so nearly attended with tragic consequence, was related when she generously presented Giles Youngs with the results of her own thorough research into the affected families.

This is a disease made elusive by reason of its various and all too often dramatic presentations. In a city where different specialties were dealt with in widely separate hospitals, victims might be considered surgical, medical, neurological or psychiatric cases, with the essential nature of the underlying disease process remaining undetected. Once recognised, the iatrogenic precipitation of acute porphyric crisis, especially by barbiturates, explains the anaesthetists' problems – and in all probability the psychiatric nurses' bewilderment at the paradoxical outcome of the attempted sedation of a 'hysterical patient'.

The recent decline in the incidence of such episodes in individuals with this form of hepatic porphyria seems likely to reflect the routine substitution of non-barbiturate sedatives. Now that genetic studies have revealed the unique status of the Chester porphyria, it is to be hoped that in the future the physician's principal role will be in counselling.

Enthusiastic cooperation between colleagues in all branches of the profession – consultants, junior and senior hospital staff, general practitioners, laboratory workers, nurses and social workers – has illuminated this fascinating research, as the ensuing chapters make plain. If the old general hospital system was still in place, and staff from all disciplines met at lunchtimes to exchange anecdotes, and perhaps, too, if we paid more attention to the naked eye study of the patient's defects before filling in the pathology request forms, instances like that described above might come to light earlier – who knows?

SIDNEY H BIRCHETT
*September 1997*

# Acknowledgements

My enjoyment in producing this monograph has been at the expense of much hard labour by many people, to all of whom I am profoundly grateful: Eunice Fletcher, Librarian, Postgraduate Medical Centre, Countess of Chester Hospital; Christine Robson and Yvonne Hughes, Chester Register Office; Simon Harrison, Chester City Public Record Office; Peter Boughton, Keeper of Art and Architecture, and Daniel Robinson, Keeper of Archaeology, Grosvenor Museum, Chester. The laboratory staff of the Chester hospitals have processed innumerable samples. In particular, Bernard Green, late Chief Biochemist, orchestrated Zorka Bekerus' endeavours. Bekerus' researches were encouraged by Geoffrey Snow, former Consultant Anaesthetist in Chester, and by Cecil Gray, former Professor of Anaesthetics in Liverpool. Only late in 1997 did I discover that Gray is still in contact with Bekerus in New York and this resulted in my first telephone conversation with her, further memorabilia and her photograph (Chapter 5).

Paul Barrow and, subsequently, Stuart Gray, Chief Executives, Countess of Chester NHS Trust, greatly facilitated the research; Wyeth Laboratories made a generous donation towards the production costs of this book; Joanne Richardson, Chief Photographer, Countess of Chester Hospital, prepared the family trees and many of the illustrations; Richard Bentall, Professor of Clinical Psychology, University of Liverpool, gave valuable statistical advice; Andrew McDonagh and Sidney Birchett improved and corrected the grammar of numerous draft manuscripts, and provided many stimulating suggestions; Professor Vivian Nutton, Wellcome Institute for the History of Medicine, advised on the historical matters in Chapter 2; Professor Sir Abraham Goldberg provided great encouragement by telephone and letter; Kenneth McColl, Goldberg's deputy for many years but now Professor of

Gastroenterology at Glasgow, has provided generous advice over the years and, with Michael Moore, helped to untangle the biochemical complexities of the Chester porphyria.

I am grateful to David Kerr (College Editor), Diana Beaven (Head of Publications) and Amanda May at the Royal College of Physicians for their support, tutelage and coordination of our efforts. I am also grateful to Mary Firth for her skilful and meticulous copy editing and to Merriton Sharp for the imaginative design of the book.

The porphobilinogen deaminase levels of the patients in the atopy study were determined in the laboratory of George Elder, Professor of Clinical Biochemistry, Cardiff. Dennis Blake and Neil Badcock tested the Australian members of the family.

Unfortunately, at the start of the project I did not grasp the nettle and master the skills of word processing and desk-top publishing. My excuse is two wonderful medical secretaries. Between 1974 and 1989, Maureen Willetts typed and retyped innumerable manuscripts without the benefit of a word processor. In retrospect, I marvel that I or any other investigator ever completed a manuscript using such basic equipment. Kathy Kusinski suffers in the opposite way – her acquisition of a word processor in 1989 has provided me with every excuse to tweak the phraseology of this monograph, sometimes the same passages several times a day. This book would not have been born without her unfailing endurance and good humour.

Our study would not have been possible without the generous cooperation of the members of the Chester porphyria family. Their illnesses have often been harrowing and both they and I have benefited from the care and commitment of nurses and junior doctors on the hospital wards. Local general practitioners have been unfailingly cooperative in allowing me to study their patients.

GRY

# Contributors

**Zorka Bekerus** MD
*Anaesthetic Registrar, Chester Hospitals (1963–65)*

**Sidney H Birchett** MB
*Medical Registrar, Chester City Hospital and Royal Infirmary (1952–56).*
*General Practitioner, Chester (1957–89)*

**David Chew** FRCP
*Medical Registrar, Chester Hospitals (1985–86).*
*Consultant Physician in Elderly Care, Chesterfield, Derbyshire*

**Roger N Chitty** FRCPsych
*Consultant Psychiatrist, Department of Liaison Psychiatry, West Cheshire Hospital, Chester*

**Susan E Church** MD, MRCP
*Medical Registrar, Chester Hospitals (1984–85).*
*Consultant Physician in Respiratory Medicine, Halton General Hospital, Runcorn, Cheshire*

**J Michael Connor** MD, DSc, FRCP
*Professor of Medical Genetics, Duncan Guthrie Institute, University of Glasgow*

**Jonathan Evans** MRCP
*Medical Registrar, Countess of Chester Hospital, Chester (1994–96)*

**Sir Abraham Goldberg** MD, DSc, FRCP, FRSE
*Emeritus Regius Professor of the Practice of Medicine, University of Glasgow*

**Terry J Kavanagh** BA
*Local Historian, Chester*

**Andrew McDonagh** FRCP
*Medical Registrar, Chester Hospitals (1988–89).*
*Consultant Dermatologist, Royal Hallamshire Hospital, Sheffield*

**Michael R Moore** BSc, PhD, DSc, MACM
*Reader in Medicine, Western Infirmary, Glasgow (1967–94).*
*Director, National Research Centre for Environmental*
*Toxicology, University of Queensland, Australia*

**Bernard Norton** MD, MRCP
*Medical Registrar, Chester Hospitals (1989–90).*
*Consultant Physician and Gastroenterologist, Derbyshire Royal*
*Infirmary, Derby*

**Colin R Porteous** FRCOG
*Obstetrics and Gynaecological Registrar, Clatterbridge Hospital*
*(1958–59).*
*Consultant Obstetrician and Gynaecologist, Southport and*
*Ormskirk Hospitals, Lancashire (1962–94)*

**Mohammad Qadiri** MRCP
*Medical Registrar, Chester Hospitals (1981–82).*
*Consultant Physician in General Medicine and Elderly Care,*
*Yeovil District Hospital, Somerset*

**Joanna Sayer** MA, MRCP
*Senior Registrar in Gastroenterology, Countess of Chester*
*Hospital, Chester (1995).*
*Specialist Registrar in Gastroenterology, John Radcliffe Hospital,*
*Oxford*

**Tudor Toma** MD
*Research Fellow, Countess of Chester Hospital, Chester (1995).*
*Resident Physician, University Medical Hospital of Iasi, Romania*

**Giles R Youngs** MD, FRCP
*Consultant Physician and Gastroenterologist, Countess of*
*Chester Hospital, Chester*

# Contents

# Historical introduction to the porphyrias

SIR ABRAHAM GOLDBERG

The porphyria diseases are mainly inborn errors of metabolism in which there are specific enzyme defects in the haem biosynthetic pathway. Haem, the iron-protoporphyrin complex, is central to biological oxidation reactions in living cells, probably contemporaneous in evolution with the emergence of life itself. In these disorders the pattern of excessive accumulation of either porphyrin precursors or formed porphyrins in the excreta or tissues relates to the location of the enzyme defect in the haem pathway (Fig 3, Chapter 12).

There are three broad clinical presentations of the porphyria diseases (the biochemical classification and the niche occupied by the Chester porphyria is discussed in Chapter 12):

1 *Acute*, with gastrointestinal and neuropsychiatric symptoms. The enzyme defect occurs prior to the formation of the tetrapyrrolic porphyrin, and the porphyrin precursor, the monopyrrole, porphobilinogen, is excreted in great excess in the urine. The most common example is acute intermittent porphyria (the highest prevalence is probably in Swedish Lapland[1]).

2 *Skin photosensitising*: the enzyme defect occurs after the formation of porphyrin, which is excreted excessively in the urine. The most common example is cutaneous hepatic porphyria (porphyria cutanea tarda).

3 *Mixed*, with both photosensitising and acute neurovisceral features, the mixture being reflected by abnormal biochemistry. The most common example is variegate porphyria (the highest prevalence is in South Africa).

## Recognition of the porphyrias as a group of diseases

Diagnosis of the porphyrias is so dependent on the chemical analysis of excreta that their historical recognition as diseases had to await the appropriate developments in chemistry. This began in 1841 when Scherer[2] added concentrated sulphuric acid to dried powdered blood and washed the precipitate free of iron. The iron-free residue was treated with alcohol which took on a blood red colour. Mülder[3] (1844) confirmed this study, and called the purple-red fluid 'iron-free haematin'. Thudicum[4] (1867) discovered the fluorescence of this material using a cone of sunlight focused by a system of quartz lenses and noted its spectrum. Hoppe-Seyler[5] (1871) renamed the substance 'haematoporphyrin'.

The scene was now set for recording in 1874 what was to be the first case diagnosed as porphyria. A 33 year old weaver had suffered skin photosensitivity since the age of three months; he had an enlarged spleen, icteric conjunctivae, and red urine containing Hoppe-Seyler's haematoporphyrin. At autopsy, his bones were coloured brown. This was undoubtedly an example of the very rare congenital erythropoietic porphyria,[6] now known to be transmitted as a Mendelian recessive character.

In 1898,[7] M'Call Anderson, at the Western Infirmary, Glasgow, described two brothers, fishermen from Stornoway, both of whom had suffered from skin photosensitivity from the age of four years and excreted haematoporphyrin in their urine. He suggested that there was a 'close connection between the cutaneous manifestations and the pigment in the urine'. This first suggestion of the photosensitising properties of porphyrins was put to the test by Meyer-Betz[8] in 1913 when he injected 200 mg of haematoporphyrin into his own veins and observed the marked photosensitising lesions on his exposed face and hands after going into the sunlight.

A few years after the introduction in 1881 of sulphonal as a hypnotic, Harley[9] reported that a young woman he treated with sulphonal in the Royal Infirmary, Edinburgh, suffered a severe nervous system disturbance with the passage of dark red urine, and died. In the same year (1890) Ranking and Pardington[10] described two women who had taken sulphonal and suffered the typical gastro-intestinal and neuropsychiatric features of what is now called 'acute intermittent porphyria'. Stokvis[11] reported a few years later that an elderly woman who had taken sulphonal excreted a dark red urine containing haematoporphyrin, and later died. In 1895, Stokvis[12] administered sulphonal to rabbits, and observed marked haematoporphyrinuria – the first example of experimental porphyria in an animal.

In the next 20 years, many other similar cases were recorded in patients who had taken sulphonal, tetronal, trional and barbiturates,[13] but also in some in whom no drug could be implicated. Today, there is a long list of drugs known to have the capacity to provoke a patient with the hereditary trait of acute porphyria into the acute form (eg alcohol, barbiturates, the contraceptive pill). These drugs have been identified over the past 100 years both by clinical observation and by experimental studies in animals.

Gunther (1911,[14] 1922[15]) classified the 'haematoporphyrinurias' into:

- *acute*,
- *congenital*, with photosensitivity from birth, and
- *chronic*, in which the photosensitivities occurred later in life.

He was also the first to recognise congenital porphyria as an 'inborn error of metabolism', the concept put forward by Garrod.[16]

## Hans Fischer's contribution

The great German chemist, Hans Fischer, of Munich, studied the porphyrin excretion of one of Gunther's patients with congenital porphyria, a man called Petry (conveniently employed by Fischer in his laboratory). When Petry died, a massive chemical and pathological investigation of his tissues was carried out, from which Fischer provided the firm foundation of porphyrin chemistry and physical properties. His synthesis of haemin was the major achievement for which he obtained the Nobel Prize in 1930.

Before the second world war Fischer's laboratory in Munich had become a Mecca for many of the major contributors to porphyria work, including Cecil Watson, of Minneapolis, Jan Waldenström, of Sweden, and Claude Rimington, of the UK. Watson, working with Fischer in 1931–32, has communicated the excitement of these years, both personally and in his remarkable *Reminiscences of Hans Fischer and his Laboratory*.[17] One of the beer-cellars that Watson visited was a favourite of the Nazi brownshirts, and he recalled seeing Hitler there before he assumed power. Waldenström, who worked in Munich in 1934–35, was a strategically placed sharp witness to Fischer's antipathy to the Nazi regime and philosophy when Rosenberg, a high-ranking Nazi, addressed the Science Faculties of Munich University in a 'command' lecture. Rosenberg ranted interminably but, amid the universal and repeated applause and stamping of feet, Fischer sat stony-faced in the middle of the front row, arms folded, immobile. Despite his known views, he managed to survive as professor of organic chemistry throughout the war until 1945 when, depressed by the damage to his laboratories, the death of many of his friends and students, and the total disruption of his research, he tragically died by his own hand. Thus, 50 years ago perished the 'man who taught us what makes blood red and grass green'.

## Porphobilinogen

On his return to Sweden from Munich, Waldenström completed his studies on the 'porphyrias', named thus instead of 'haematoporphyrias'. His valuable contributions included a clinical survey of 103 Swedish cases of acute porphyria, published in 1937.[18] There was a dense clustering of cases in Northern Lapland, and Waldenström's numerous family trees emphasised that the disease was transmitted as a Mendelian dominant character. Harley had noted in 1890[9] that his patients' urine contained a chromogen which darkened on standing to form 'haematoporphyrin'. Paula Sachs discovered in 1931[19] that the urine in acute cases contained a substance which, on the addition of Ehrlich's aldehyde reagent, gave a red colour insoluble in chloroform, and was therefore not urobilinogen. Waldenström and Vahlquist[20] named this 'porphobilinogen'. This compound was shown 20 years later in Rimington's laboratory to be the essential monopyrrolic precursor of the porphyrins.[21] Using Ehrlich's aldehyde test for porphobilinogen, Waldenström found that it was sometimes positive in asymptomatic siblings and second- and third-generation relatives of patients with the active disease, so he named this group 'latent porphyria'. The porphobilinogen test also proved to be a rapid and useful method of confirming or refuting a suspected diagnosis.

## Neuropathological changes and clinical features of the porphyrias

A clinical study in the UK[22] of 50 cases of acute porphyria showed a similar pattern to that in Sweden, and emphasised the association of barbiturates with the paralytic features. Schmid *et al* stressed in 1954[23] that the liver was the predominant site of the metabolic dyscrasia in acute porphyria – this became apparent in the various experimental animal types of porphyria mimicking the acute disease in man.[24,25] Despite the uncanny chemical replication of acute porphyria in rabbits, rats and fowls with the non-hypnotic allylisopropyl acetamide, the clinical features of the human disease were not observed,[25] confirming the absence of pharmacological activity in studies on porphyrins and porphobilinogen.[26] There are postmortem neuropathological changes in the central nervous system, peripheral and autonomic nerves which can explain all the clinical features of the acute disease.[22,27] Nearly 40 years after this observation, the exact relationship between the disorder of haem synthesis and the neuropathological changes remains an enigma. It still seems a reasonable hypothesis that a haem deficiency of neural tissue affecting tissue oxidation is involved.[22,28]

## Chester porphyria

The understanding of the porphyrias has been made possible by chemical and biochemical advances, together with observations by numerous clinicians throughout the world. Biochemical developments by Rimington and others simplifying the accurate testing of porphyrins in excreta have facilitated extensive studies of known types of porphyria throughout the world, as well as identifying new types. Unlocking the secrets of hereditary disorders requires the intellectual bravura of a Sherlock Holmes and the pertinacity of a Professor Moriarty. This formula was clearly operative in the elucidation of Chester porphyria by Giles Youngs and his colleagues.

Chester porphyria reflects authentically the clinical picture of acute intermittent porphyria, but its haem enzyme defects (in porphobilinogen deaminase and protoporphyrinogen oxidase) and excretory anomalies of porphyrin metabolism bestride the two separate disorders of acute intermittent porphyria and variegate porphyria. No skin features have been observed. Thus, over the past 30 years a biochemically unique type of porphyria has been identified, ostensibly occasioned by a marital union in Chester about 100 years ago. The ancient, beautiful walled city of Chester, dating back to the Roman occupation, was therefore the crucible for the generation and multiplication of a unique disorder.

The Chester team has used its clinical skills to the full, and has also collaborated with experts in different fields: biochemists, geneticists, general practitioners, nursing staff and social workers. All this has contributed to the health of the community, not just to the porphyric families, because a work of this quality projects a paradigm for others to follow.

There are other lessons too. There is still – and always will be – a place for clinical observation and for listening to the patient and his or her relatives. Amid the controversies surrounding the National Health Service, the need to foster clinical research must not be underestimated. Each time a doctor prescribes a drug represents an experiment; although the drug's effects are well-known, the idiosyncrasies of the patient may be hidden. This is well illustrated by the astute anaesthetist Zorka Bekerus who, in 1963, diagnosed a porphyric crisis when a patient in Chester collapsed on induction of anaesthesia with thiopentone – an observation which started the saga of the Chester porphyria.

Therapeutics may be the last to profit from scientific research – the ailing beggar seeking crumbs from the rich man's table – but without that research the chance of successful treatment in hereditary disorders is not much greater than that of the medieval alchemist in his chemical kitchen striving to transmute base metal into gold. Elegant studies from Michael Connor's laboratory in Glasgow,[29] in association with Youngs' group, have pinpointed the genetic locus of Chester porphyria to chromosome 11q, but at a different site from porphobilinogen deaminase, thus both differentiating it from acute intermittent porphyria and confirming the uniqueness of the disease. Moreover, this is the first step towards cloning the gene for Chester porphyria, and could well contribute to future treatment in the form of gene therapy, of which we have already witnessed the dawn elsewhere.[30]

# References

1 Andersson C (ed). *Acute intermittent porphyria in northern Sweden. A population-based study*. Umeå University Medical Dissertations, New Series No. 497. Umeå and Arjeplog, Sweden: University of Umeå and Primary Health Care Centre, Arjeplog, 1997.

2 Scherer J. Untersuchungen Liebigs. *Annalen der Chemie und Pharmacie* 1841; **40**: 1–64.

3 Mülder GH. Über eisenfreis Hämatin. *Jahrbuch für Praktische Chemie* 1844; **32**: 186–97.

4 Thudicum JLW. *Report on researches intended to promote an improved chemical identification of disease*. 10th report of the medical officer, Privy Council, Appendix 7. London: HMSO, 1867: 152–95, 200, 227–33.

5 Hoppe-Seyler F. Das Hämatin Tübinger Med-Chem. *Untersuchungen* 1871; **4**: 523–33.

6 Schultz JH. *Ein Fall von Pemphigus Leprosus, kompliziert durch lepra visceralis*. Inaugural dissertation, Greifswald, 1874.

7 M'Call Anderson T. Hydroa aestivale in two brothers, complicated with the presence of haematoporphyrin in the urine. *British Journal of Dermatology* 1898; **10**: 1–4.

8 Meyer-Betz F. Untersuchungen Über die Biologische (photodynamische) Wirkung des Haematoporphyrins und anderen Derivate des Blut und Gallenfarbstoffs. *Deutsches Archiv für Klinische Medizin* 1913; **112**: 476–503.

9  Harley V. Two fatal cases of an unusual form of nerve disturbance associated with dark-red urine, probably due to defective tissue oxidation. *British Medical Journal* 1890; **2**: 1169–70.

10  Ranking JE, Pardington GL. Two cases of haemato-porphyrin in the urine. *Lancet* 1890; **ii**: 607–9.

11  Stokvis BJ. Over Twee Zeldsame Kleurstoffen in Urine van Zicken. *Nederlands Tijdschrift voor Geneeskunde (Amsterdam)* 1889; **13**: 409–17.

12  Stokvis BJ. Zur pathogenese der Hamatoporphyrinurie. *Zeitschrift fuer Klinische Medizin* 1895; **28**: 1–21.

13  Dobrschansky M. Einiges über Malonal. *Wiener Medizinische Presse* 1906; **47**: 2145.

14  Gunther H. Die Haematoporphyrie. *Deutsche Archiv für Klinische Medizin* 1912; **105**: 89–146.

15  Gunther H. Die Bedeutung der Haematoporphyrinurie in der Physiologie und Pathologie. *Ergebnisse Allgemeinen Pathologie und Pathologischen Anatomie* 1922; **20**: 608–764.

16  Garrod AE. *Inborn errors of metabolism*, 2nd edn. London: H Frowde, 1923.

17  Watson CJ. Reminiscences of Hans Fischer and his laboratory. *Perspectives in Biology and Medicine* 1965; **8**: 419–35.

18  Waldenström J. Studien über porphyrie. *Acta Medica Scandinavica* 1937; **92** (Suppl 82): 1–254.

19  Sachs P. Ein Fall von akuter Porphyrie mit hochgradiger Muskelatrophie. *Klinische Wochenschrift* 1931; **10**: 1123–5.

20  Waldenström J, Vahlquist BC. Studien über die Enstehung der roten Harnpigmente (Uroporphyrin und Porphobilin) bei der akuten Porphyrie aus ihrer farblosen Vorstufe (Porphobilinogen). *Zeitschrift für Physiologische Chemie (Hoppe-Seyler)* 1939; **260**: 189–209.

21  Falk JE, Dresel EIB, Rimington C. Porphobilinogen as porphyrin precursor, and interconversion of porphyrins in a tissue system. *Nature* 1953; **172**: 292–4.

22  Goldberg A. Acute intermittent porphyria. A study of 50 cases. *Quarterly Journal of Medicine* 1959; NS **28**: 183–209.

23  Schmid R, Schwartz S, Watson CJ. Porphyrin content of bone marrow and liver in the various forms of porphyria. *Archives of Internal Medicine* 1954; **93**: 167–90.

24  Schmid R, Schwartz S. Experimental porphyria. III. Hepatic type produced by sedormid. *Proceedings of the Society for Experimental Biology and Medicine* 1952; **81**: 685–9.

25  Goldberg A, Rimington C. Experimentally produced porphyria in animals. *Proceedings of the Royal Society of London, Series B* 1955; **143**: 257–80.

26  Goldberg A, Paton WDM, Thompson JW. Pharmacology of the porphyrins and porphobilinogen. *British Journal of Pharmacology* 1954; **9**: 91–4.

27  Gibson JB, Goldberg A. The neuropathology of acute porphyria. *Journal of Pathology and Bacteriology* 1956; **71**: 495–509.

28 Yeung Laiwah AC, Moore MR, Goldberg A. Pathogenesis of acute porphyria. *Quarterly Journal of Medicine* 1987; **63**: 377–92.

29 Norton B, Lanyon WG, Moore MR, Porteous M, *et al.* Evidence for involvement of a second genetic locus on chromosome 11q in porphyrin metabolism. *Human Genetics* 1993; **91**: 576–8.

30 Culver KW. *Gene therapy. A handbook for physicians*. New York: Mary Ann Liebert Inc, 1994.

*Part 1*

# The origins of porphyria in Chester

*Chapter 1*

# The story of the Chester porphyria kindred

GILES YOUNGS

I have always found the biochemical and classification aspects of porphyria difficult to master, but we are fortunate that the disease has an evocative name, 'porphyria', derived from the Greek *porphuros* (or purple), a reference to the coloured urine passed by affected subjects. Awareness of the condition has recently been enhanced by the appellation 'The Royal Malady' as the explanation for King George III's scourge, and publicised by Alan Bennett's play and film *The Madness of King George III*.[1] This renown is far removed from the circumstances of the large Chester family whose history I wish to relate. It will be described later how this family arose among a quarrelsome community of salmon fishermen on the River Dee. Many of their number died at a young age from a cause unrecognised by their medical practitioners, but shown by our study to be porphyria.

The acute hepatic porphyrias are a group of conditions caused by a dominantly inherited deficiency of one or other of the enzymes involved in the synthesis of haem. For reasons unknown to medical science, only some people inheriting the deficiency develop symptoms (abdominal and limb pains, peripheral neuropathy and psychiatric disturbance). Manifestations occur in attacks, which are sometimes fatal and often, but not always, precipitated by prescribed medication, particularly barbiturates. The presenting symptoms are often bizarre; they can mimic other more common conditions reminiscent of that other notorious hoaxer, syphilis, so that Waldenström applied to porphyria the epithet *la petite simulatrice*[2] (as opposed to syphilis, 'the big simulator'). This explains why mistaken diagnoses have been made and incorrect death certificates issued in the Chester porphyria family.[3,4] Not surprisingly,

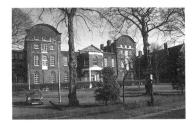

**Fig 1**. Chester Royal Infirmary (opened 1755, closed 1996).

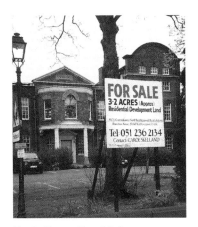

**Fig 2**. Chester Royal Infirmary today – for sale.

the patients' medical advisers were diagnostically perplexed, thus creating a recipe for inappropriate management, misunderstanding, and a suspicion of hysteria or malingering. The doctors' performance was further tarnished in the eyes of their patients by a lack of awareness of the long-term sequelae of porphyria – chronic hypertension and renal failure – little reported in the literature but common in porphyric members of the Chester kindred.

## The beginning of my interest in porphyria

My interest in porphyria started in 1980 with an unpleasant outpatient consultation at the Chester Royal Infirmary (Fig 1), now sadly closed (Fig 2). The mother of my patient (a 16 year old girl, notation 1.6.5.3*) quickly surmised that I had never seen a case of porphyria. Before taking the family history, I judged it necessary to allay obvious anxieties with platitudes about the benign prognosis of porphyria – whereupon the mother told me that four years earlier both her husband (1.6.5), aged 38, and her son (1.6.5.1), aged 17, had died of porphyria within six months of each other. A year later, her husband's sister died of renal complications of porphyria. Eleven of her husband's cousins (1.1.1, 1.1.5, 1.2.1, 1.2.3, 1.2.4, 1.2.8, 1.5.1, 1.5.3, 1.7.1, 1.9.1, 1.9.3) had died, nine of them aged 40 years or less. Although porphyria was mentioned on the death certificate of only two of these (1.1.5, 1.9.3), the family suspected a common theme, especially as five died with paralysis. I was rightly accused of being as ignorant of the condition as all the other local hospital and general practitioners (GPs).

Stung by her condemnation, and further motivated by the frequent admissions of my patient with acute porphyric crises (Chapter 7), I resolved to study the family. I was greatly helped in this by the enthusiasm of my medical registrar, Mohammad Qadiri, a Palestinian who had qualified in Baghdad and come to this country for further training. Our patient's mother provided the names and addresses of her late husband's siblings – and so Qadiri's quest began. The eldest sibling, 1.6.1 (our patient's uncle), was and continues to be a fount of information, and we are deeply indebted to him. He had suffered porphyric crises as a young man, and limited his family to one child because of the premature deaths of his young cousins from what he guessed was the same condition. We show in Chapter 6 that his suspicion was almost certainly correct.

## The search begins

Qadiri held an onerous clinical post as one of only two registrars looking after 120 acute medical beds at the Chester City Hospital,

---

*For an explanation of the notation, refer to the glossary at the end of the book.

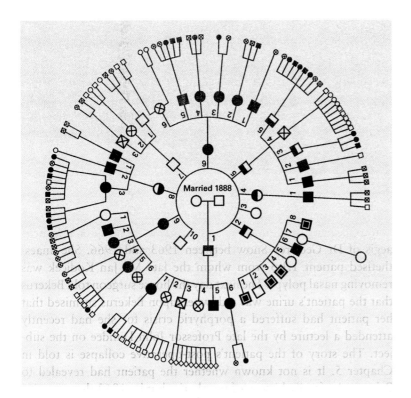

Fig 3. The Chester porphyria pedigree
(1995) (updated from Ref 4)
(circles = female; squares = male)
▬ = obligatory porphyria;
■ = porphyria biochemistry-positive;
⊠ = porphyria biochemistry-negative;
▣ = porphyria-positive, history only;
□ = not tested;
◇ = unknown sex.

and his need to learn gastrointestinal endoscopy surpassed any requirement for research. Nevertheless, he spent his evenings driving around Chester searching for members of the kindred in order to construct a family tree (Fig 3). His information was often vague: 'look for a brown mini parked outside the house towards the end of the street', or 'try the butcher's shop two streets along'. He quickly learned that the family was large (38 cousins), only three of whom had migrated from Chester. More amazingly, he learnt that he was not the first 'foreign doctor' to knock on doors unannounced seeking personal and medical information, some of which aroused unhappy memories and sometimes hostile emotions. The family members were only too well aware of the deaths of several of their number at a young age, and that illnesses were often complicated by epilepsy (Chapter 7) and admission to the County Mental Hospital (Chapter 11). Qadiri became aware of mistrust of the medical profession: family members had died unexpectedly after bizarre illnesses (Chapter 6), their complaints of abdominal pain had been fobbed off, hysteria was often suspected (Chapter 11) and paralysis unexplained. He found that some of them denied that the taint affected their line, despite obvious evidence to the contrary.

Qadiri's enthusiasm might easily have been dampened in this unpromising setting, and he was not helped by the ambience in the

13

endoscopy suite, the venue he usually chose to update me on his researches. Just as it is difficult to hold a conversation while watching a television programme so it is with endoscopy, and I often found myself only half listening. His fortitude overcame all this; moreover, his detective work with the family members was greatly helped by the unforeseen blessing that the 'foreign doctor' who had preceded him was held in high esteem and remembered with affection.

## The contribution of Zorka Bekerus

Zorka Bekerus was a Yugoslavian anaesthetic registrar, working at the Chester Royal Infirmary and Barrowmore Hospital under the aegis of Dr Geoffrey Snow between 1963 and 1966. She anaesthetised patient 1.1.5 from whom the late Mr Jan Kodicek was removing nasal polyps. The next day the house surgeon told Bekerus that the patient's urine was red, whereupon Bekerus surmised that her patient had suffered a porphyric crisis for she had recently attended a lecture by the late Professor John Dundee on the subject. The story of the patient's post-operative collapse is told in Chapter 5. It is not known whether the patient had revealed to Bekerus the family history of porphyria, but by 1963 three cousins (1.6.3, 1.6.5, 1.9.3) had been diagnosed. The first two, although Chester residents, were under the care of Clatterbridge Hospital 12 miles away, and the third had died of respiratory paralysis at the Chester City Hospital in 1958, aged 22 years. There was thus no current interest in porphyria in Chester.

Bekerus's researches are well remembered by colleagues and family members alike. She visited numerous families in their homes and collected repeated urine and occasional stool samples. By the time Qadiri and I began our enquiries in 1980, the trail pioneered by Bekerus had become indistinct. She went to London in about 1966 and then to the USA. None of her records was extant, but many family members had been told their porphyria status, and occasional copies of letters from Bekerus informing patients of this were found in their hospital case-notes (Fig 4). She subsequently received anxious enquiries from members after she left Chester (see Appendix for examples).

Over the next nine years I consulted relevant directories and specialist anaesthetic societies in the USA in the hope of tracing Bekerus, then suddenly in 1989 I was delighted to receive a large package labelled 'extremely urgent, please rush to addressee'! The contents fulfilled my hopes: out tumbled documents prepared

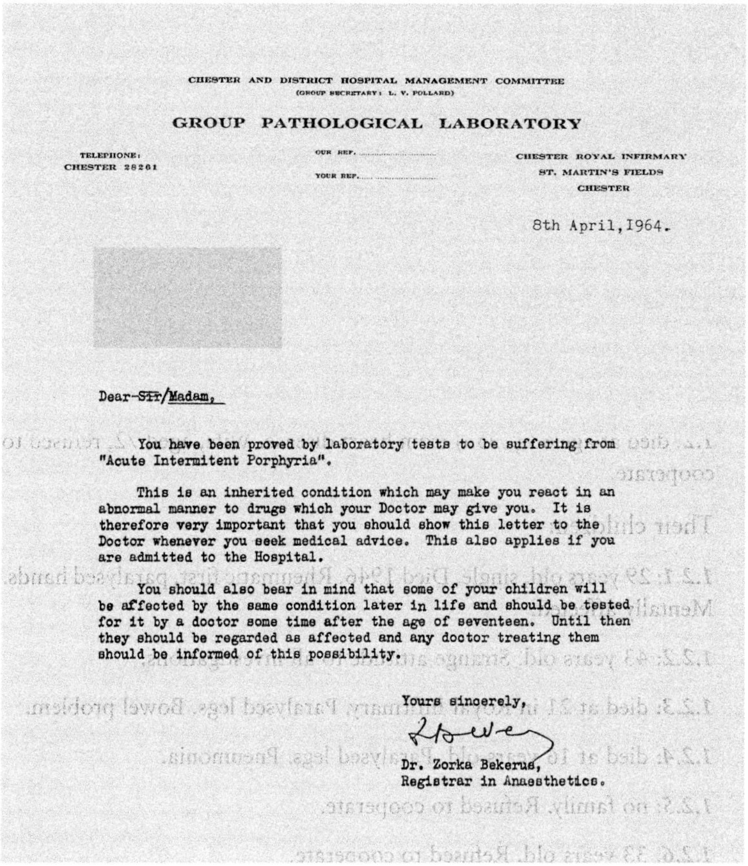

CHESTER AND DISTRICT HOSPITAL MANAGEMENT COMMITTEE
(GROUP SECRETARY: L. V. POLLARD)

**GROUP PATHOLOGICAL LABORATORY**

TELEPHONE:
CHESTER 25261

OUR REF. ................

YOUR REF. ................

CHESTER ROYAL INFIRMARY
ST. MARTIN'S FIELDS
CHESTER

8th April, 1964.

Dear ~~Sir~~/Madam,

You have been proved by laboratory tests to be suffering from "Acute Intermittent Porphyria".

This is an inherited condition which may make you react in an abnormal manner to drugs which your Doctor may give you. It is therefore very important that you should show this letter to the Doctor whenever you seek medical advice. This also applies if you are admitted to the Hospital.

You should also bear in mind that some of your children will be affected by the same condition later in life and should be tested for it by a doctor some time after the age of seventeen. Until then they should be regarded as affected and any doctor treating them should be informed of this possibility.

Yours sincerely,

Dr. Zorka Bekerus,
Registrar in Anaesthetics.

Fig 4. Letter from Dr Bekerus advising subject 1.9 of her positive porphyria status.

25 years earlier, a draft unpublished manuscript (which forms Chapter 5), a family tree (Fig 4, Chapter 5), and biographical notes – all of which were valuable additions to our existing records.

Bekerus had made notes on all members of the families visited, including the children, and referred to urine testing for porphobilinogen, the occurrence of paralysis, hypertension and mental illness. Her notes also mirror the daily vicissitudes of life, which perhaps afflict the members of the porphyric kindred more than most. Some extracts are given here*:

*Girl*: died aged two years old on father's knee [no notation as died young].

*1.1.6.1*: 6½ years old. Bronchitis at three years old, developed to bronchial asthma. Constipation as baby and hard stools. Red hair and freckles.

*1.3.1.5*: 12 years old. Not very intelligent. Small for his age. Glasses. Inherited short sight from mother.

---

*The extracts are verbatim except for minor editorial changes and the addition of the modern family notation.

15

*1.5.1*: 43 years old. In Deva Hospital (County Mental Hospital). Strange. Wife divorced him. Stubborn. Urine was negative until GP loaded him with barbiturates.

*1.5.2*: 40 years old. Married, and wife left him after first night. Bad temper, headaches. Refused to have urine test. February 1965, admitted to Deva Hospital. GP treated him with barbiturates, and urine became positive.

*1.8.1*: 35 years old. Negative past history but in April had nervous exhaustion, took something for nerves, and urine became positive.

The biographical notes on the family of one member, 1.2, starkly illustrate the tragedy and pathos of the kindred:

*1.2*: died at age 63 (1953) from heart disease. Wife, aged 72, refused to cooperate.

Their children:

*1.2.1*: 29 years old, single. Died 1946. Rheumatic first, paralysed hands. Mentally affected.

*1.2.2*: 43 years old. Strange attitude to all investigations.

*1.2.3*: died at 21 in Royal Infirmary. Paralysed legs. Bowel problem.

*1.2.4*: died at 16 years old. Paralysed legs. Pneumonia.

*1.2.5*: no family. Refused to cooperate.

*1.2.6*: 33 years old. Refused to cooperate.

*1.2.7*: 29 years old. One child. Refused to cooperate.

*1.2.8*: died 18 years old (1951). Appendicitis operation and, after one year, back in City Hospital, died in one month's time. At the end was paralysed and confused.

Thus, four of the eight siblings died between the ages of 16 and 29 years. Their respective death certificates (Chapter 6) record:

- uraemia, nephritis and mental deficiency;
- myotonia atrophica;
- pneumonia, operation and appendicitis; and
- left ventricular failure and malignant hypertension.

An examination of these death certificates 40 years later show that they were incomplete, the brothers' varying terminal illnesses almost certainly being manifestations of acute hepatic porphyria. The three remaining siblings and their mother refused to cooperate with Bekerus – perhaps by this time they had become disillusioned with their medical advisers.

Bekerus acknowledges that at the start of her study two family members were known to have porphyria but, surprisingly, does not reveal their identity in her biographical notes or in the text of her draft manuscript (Chapter 5). By 1989, when her documents arrived, it was already known from our own researches that three cousins of her index case had been diagnosed at the time of Bekerus' study in 1963:

*1.6.3*: diagnosed in 1954 when psychosis and complete paralysis complicated treatment (almost certainly barbiturates) for malignant hypertension (Chapter 4); transferred from the County Mental Hospital in Chester to a neurological bed in Clatterbridge Hospital.

*1.6.5*: her brother, aged 20, discharged from the army in 1958 because of epileptic fits; developed abdominal pains and vomiting after being given phenobarbitone; investigated at Clatterbridge Hospital and diagnosed to have porphyria (Chapter 6).

*1.9.3*: their cousin, died aged 22 years at Chester City Hospital of respiratory paralysis; her death certificate was the first to report porphyria (Table 3, Chapter 6).

It is uncertain how many of these events were known to Bekerus and it is strange that she was aware of only two of the three cases, both of which were known to the late Dr AC Hughes, physician at the Chester City Hospital, under whose care the third case, 1.9.3, died in 1958. The Clatterbridge physicians wrote to him in 1958 seeking information, to which he replied giving details of case 1.9.3 and expressing interest in the family. Bekerus certainly knew of subject 1.6.5 because her biographical notes refer to his army records. We can only surmise that Bekerus did not gain access to the Clatterbridge – and possibly the Chester City Hospital – case-notes of the three subjects.

Whatever the explanation, the contribution Bekerus made to the Chester porphyria story is pivotal: she constructed a complete family tree (Fig 4, Chapter 5), and her attribution of porphyric status to the family members is impressively similar to the modern version (Fig 3). Remarkably, on the basis of urine and faecal studies, she suggested that the Chester porphyria was typical of neither acute intermittent nor variegate porphyria (Chapter 5). Above all, she took a sympathetic interest in the family, so that many members felt that their woes had been heeded at last. Unfortunately, no clinician took up her mantle after she left Chester in 1966 until my interest began in 1980. During these 14 years, seven family members (1.9, 1.1.1, 1.1.5, 1.6.3, 1.6.5, 1.6.5.1, 1.8.3.3) died of porphyria or the complications thereof (Chapter 6).

### Diagnosis of porphyria in the index patient (1.6.3)

Having lauded the endeavours of Bekerus and Qadiri, to whom is the accolade of primogenital diagnosis of subject 1.6.3 in 1954 to be given? The patient's story is described in Chapter 4. The medical records from the Chester City Hospital and the County Mental Hospital are incomplete, but fortunately Clatterbridge Hospital records were microfilmed and are available. On being admitted with abdominal symptoms, renal failure and malignant hypertension, patient 1.6.3 was seen in the Chester City Hospital by two consultant physicians, Dr AC Hughes and the late Dr GA Kiloh. She became psychotic (probably because of barbiturate administration) and was transferred to the County Mental Hospital under the care of Dr Dewi Jones. After developing a complete flaccid paralysis, she was moved to a neurological bed at Clatterbridge Hospital under the care of the consultant neurologist, the late Dr RR Hughes.

The first mention of porphyria was in two documents, both dated 14 October 1954:

1 The referral letter from the Senior Psychiatric Registrar at the County Mental Hospital, Dr NP Langsten, to Clatterbridge, giving porphyria and polyarteritis nodosa as the differential diagnosis.

2 The clerking notes at Clatterbridge by Dr AG Shaper, Registrar to Dr RR Hughes, which concluded that:

*this patient has porphyria probably precipitated by barbiturates given for sedation when in mental home.*

The contents of Dr Langsten's letter suggests that the possibility of porphyria was first mooted at the County Mental Hospital by him or Dr Dewi Jones, or following a visiting consultation by Dr RR Hughes, or in a telephone conversation with either Dr RR Hughes or Dr Shaper requesting an opinion or transfer of the patient because of her paralysis. The relevant records are not extant, but from my questioning of some of the people involved it is clear that porphyria was Dr Shaper's diagnosis. He was almost uniquely placed to do this because not long before he had been a medical student with Professor Lennox Eales at Groote Schuur Hospital in Cape Town. This was the decade when the clinical aspects of acute porphyria were put on the map by Geoffrey Dean and Lennox Eales in South Africa, and by Abraham Goldberg in the UK. The pioneers of the biochemical and classification aspects of porphyria, most notably Fischer, Waldenström and Rimington, are described in the historical survey by Goldberg.

Early in my interest in the Chester porphyria, I became aware of Dr CR Porteous' report of case 1.6.3 in an obstetric journal,[5] but it was only in 1995 that I traced Dr Shaper and was intrigued to find that he presaged all subsequent research by including a description of subject 1.6.3 in a review article in the *Central African Journal of Medicine* in 1958.[6] The story remains as fascinating today (Chapter 4). The choice of journal meant that the publication was not picked up by the standard methods of literature searching. Dr Shaper (retired Professor of Epidemiology at the Royal Free Hospital School of Medicine, London) remembers case 1.6.3 well more than 40 years after caring for her. He modestly declined to share authorship of Chapter 4 with Dr Porteous and me. It has proved impossible to trace Dr Langsten (his name does not appear in contemporary editions of either the Medical Directory or the Medical Register), while Dr RR Hughes died in 1991.

## Genetic studies

A further piece of the jigsaw puzzle was completed by Drs Kenneth McColl and Michael Moore working in Professor Goldberg's unit in Glasgow. From 1981, but particularly in 1984 when Dr Susan Church was my medical registrar in Chester, we sent our Glasgow colleagues numerous blood, urine and faecal specimens. It became apparent that there was something peculiar about the pattern of the porphyrin excretion products. Some subjects' urine and faecal results were in keeping with acute intermittent porphyria, others with variegate porphyria, while some had an intermediate pattern (Chapter 12). This strange mixed, or dual, porphyria had scarcely been recognised hitherto in the porphyria literature. Unbeknown to us at the time, Bekerus had made the same observation 20 years before (Chapter 5). Partial elucidation came in two stages. McColl and Moore found that members of the Chester porphyria family had an unusual dual enzyme deficiency both of porphobilinogen deaminase (reduced in acute intermittent porphyria) and of protoporphyrinogen oxidase (reduced in variegate porphyria)[7] (Chapter 12).

How could this be explained if the adage 'one gene, one enzyme' is to be believed? Could it be, by exquisite chance, that two people each with a rare disease had married and the genes thereafter had been co-inherited? This seemed unlikely as it would imply the genes lying close together on the same chromosome, whereas the gene for acute intermittent porphyria was known to be on chromosome 11,[8] and the gene for variegate porphyria was believed to lie on

19

chromosome 14.[9] Some clarification came in 1989 when, this time under the aegis of my medical registrar, Bernard Norton, a further surge of samples from Chester to Glasgow was directed to Professor Michael Connor's medical genetic laboratory where they were frozen pending Norton's arrival, accompanied by his wife and two infants in the middle of a Glaswegian winter. Norton defrosted the samples, and subjected them to scientific scrutiny in the warmth of the laboratory while – as if illustrating the zero'th law of thermodynamics – his family froze in a scarcely heated bedsit, all that his meagre grant afforded. Whether the end justified the means depends on which party is asked! Norton confirmed the apparent uniqueness of the Chester porphyria by demonstrating that the gene lies on chromosome 11q, at a site different from that of acute intermittent porphyria.[10,11]

The task is not finished: the gene has not been cloned, and it is unknown why subjects have the dual enzyme deficiency. It seems that there is more to be learnt about the mechanics of haem synthesis, and that unravelling the mysteries of the Chester porphyria may help illuminate this process so essential to the evolution of the animal kingdom.

## Other symptoms of Chester porphyria

Meanwhile, my fascination with the Chester porphyria focused on less esoteric matters, helped by the zeal of two more medical registrars. We had noted the high morbidity and mortality from hypertension, cerebrovascular accident and chronic renal failure in the kindred[4] (Chapters 6 and 7), and Susan Church confirmed this in a retrospective and prospective study (Chapter 8).[12,13] She hoped her data would help us adjudicate between two rival theories about porphyria:

- that the kidney is in some way damaged, and the humoral consequences cause hypertension, or
- that the hypertension comes first, and then damages the kidney.

I leave the reader to judge, after perusing Chapter 8, whether the experiences of the Chester porphyria family members have made any contribution towards solving the above conundrum.

A second fascination for me was the high prevalence of symptomatic and often fatal porphyria in a surprisingly large proportion of the kindred. Not only were 24 of 38 cousins (63%) carriers of the gene, compared with the 25% expected by Mendelian law, but 18 of the 24 (75%) were symptomatic (Table 2, Chapter 7), in contrast to Goldberg's Scottish series[14] in which the vast majority of patients with the genetic trait for acute intermittent porphyria were clinically latent and never manifested porphyric symptoms. There was also a male preponderance of symptomatic porphyria in contradistinction to other series.

## Genealogy of the family

Further work on the family tree became mandatory, especially as one explanation for the high prevalence of porphyria in the family was a consanguineous marriage. My medical registrar in 1987, Andrew McDonagh, became the genealogist to the pedigree. He visited churches, graveyards and the Chester Public Record Office, and was able to trace the lineage to the late 18th century. His views on the likelihood of a consanguineous marriage are expressed in Chapter 3. Qadiri and I think such a union quite likely, but McDonagh is much more cautious. When I spoke to a local medical audience about 10 years ago using the rather pompous Latinised title *porphyria cestriensis*, a local GP, Dr Austen Elliott, suggested an alternative epithet for the complaint, *porphyria incestuensis!*

Not only have 16 of the 24 porphyric grandchildren died, compared with only one of their nine non-porphyric cousins (Chapter 6), but some had incorrect diagnoses and death certificates (Chapters 6 and 7), with the true cause of their painful and distressing illnesses unrecognised. This is best exemplified by considering the high prevalence of psychiatric illness in the porphyric, but not the non-porphyric, members of the family, complications well recognised in the literature and in Alan Bennett's *The Madness of King George III*.[1] It is much disputed by the pundits whether there is such an entity as a 'porphyric personality'. Roger Chitty attempts to answer the question for the Chester family in Chapter 11.

## Peter Dobson, the first case of Chester porphyria

Peter Dobson was born in 1867 into a community of salmon fishermen living in Stye or Sty Lane (later renamed Greenway Street) in the Handbridge district of Chester, on the west bank of the River Dee which runs through the city, and reached from the city by crossing the medieval Old Dee Bridge (Fig 5). Stye Lane is shown both on Stockdale's map of 1796 (Fig 6) and on John Speed's map of 1610. A little of the colourful way of life of the fisher-folk, including their privations and rather frequent visits to the magistrate's court, is described in Chapter 3.

Peter Dobson was one of three illegitimate children, and so took his mother's surname – according to the *Chester Chronicle*, she was

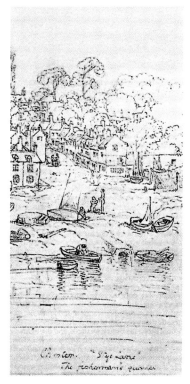

**Fig 5.** Stye Lane (Greenway Street), Chester, 1850 (anonymous sketch) – 'the fishermen's quarter'.

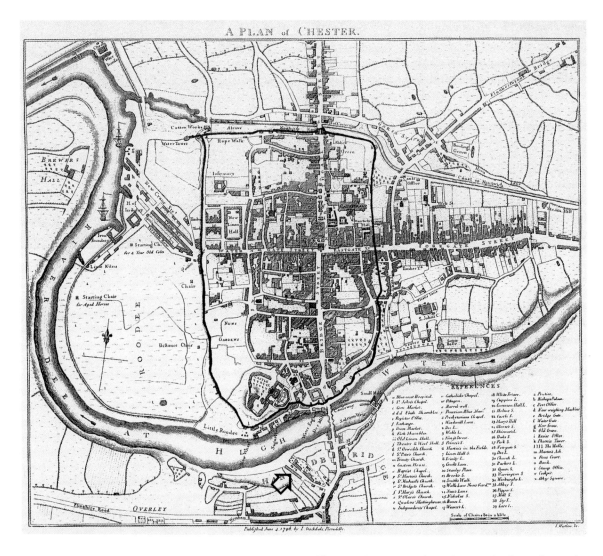

**Fig 6.** Stockdale's map of Chester, 1796. The arrow (⟲) shows Stye Lane (Greenway Street). The cruciform main streets and encircling city wall date from Roman times (Chapter 2). The infirmary lies within the north-west corner of the walls.

a prostitute (see Chapter 3). It was he who might have been the product of a consanguineous union. He married Sarah Pay in 1888 and had 14 children. Seven of the 10 who survived into adult life had porphyria, and there is circumstantial evidence to suggest that more – or even all – of the siblings may have been porphyric (Chapters 3 and 6). An abbreviated family tree (Fig 7) shows that 58 of the 106 great-grandchildren (generation IV) are at risk of porphyria because they have a porphyric parent; 48 of them have been tested and 25 of them have porphyria. The parental status of 52 of the great-grandchildren is known: 10 have no children, and the remaining 42 have 86 children to date. If the fecundity of the great-grandchildren of unknown parental status is similar, there are currently about 175 great-great-grandchildren (generation V). There are already 10 great-great-great grandchildren (generation VI). Thus, Peter and Sarah Dobson presently have over 330 descendants. This is a fecundity reminiscent of the one million living Afrikaners who bear the family names of 20 of the original Dutch settlers,[15] many of whom carry the gene for variegate porphyria[16] and so illustrate Malthusian law.

In addition to its fecundity, the family is characterised by its low migration rate: only three of the 38 grandchildren have left Chester. It is ironic that a century earlier the eminent Chester physician, John Haygarth (Chapter 2), lamented the small number of children per marriage in the city.[17] Our family is the second largest with porphyria to be reported in the UK, Andrews *et al* having described a kindred of 414 in Plymouth with hereditary coproporphyria.[18]

The manifestations of porphyria are protean, and other illnesses are often mimicked which, as explained earlier, is why the epithet *la petite simulatrice* was used by Waldenström in one of his many seminal papers on acute porphyria.[2] This symptomatic mimicry explains many of the incorrect diagnoses and death certificates (Chapters 6 and 7). Recognition by the medical profession in Chester of the personal tragedies suffered in the family was additionally delayed because family members presented with their porphyric symptoms to many different GPs, physicians, surgeons, psychiatrists, gynaecologists and anaesthetists (Table 1, Chapter 7) at any of the four Chester hospitals – all on different sites, although under the same health authority.

## Dobson's complaint

Family members have long been aware of their affliction. Some lost confidence in their physicians, who gave them a variety of contradictory diagnoses and explanations, especially those who encountered doctors' disbelief in their widespread pains, curious pareses, and emotional disturbances accompanied by only vague physical signs and normal investigations (see Appendix). Nine have died of porphyria aged 30 years or less, including four brothers. One patient told his GP that he suffered with 'Dobson's complaint' – the family name, and hence incorporated in the title of this monograph (Fig 8). The large South African kindred with variegate porphyria described by Geoffrey Dean[16] illustrates the same tragedies and pathos. Members of that kindred also presaged recognition by the medical profession by coining the sobriquet for their family affliction 'van Rooyen's skin'.

The five decades 1940–90 span the young adult and middle life of the 38 Chester grandchildren, many of whom suffered or died

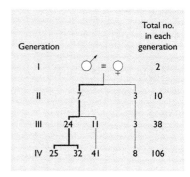

**Fig 7.** Abbreviated family tree of kindred showing numbers in each generation with porphyria (thick lines, heavy type: porphyria-positive subjects; light type: negative or untested subjects). It is estimated that there are currently about 175 members of generation V, and there are known to be 10 members of generation VI.

23

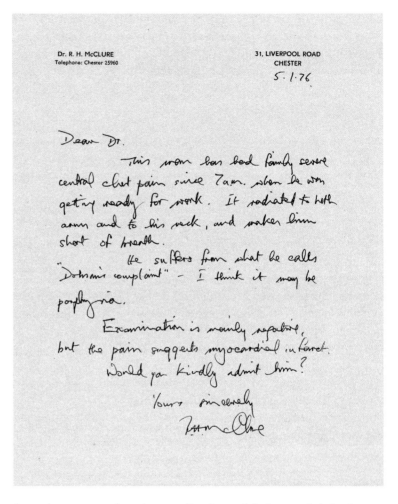

**Fig 8.** Extract from Dr R McClure's letter mentioning that subject 1.5.2 has 'Dobson's complaint'.

from the acute or chronic complications of their genetic inheritance. Not surprisingly, barbiturates played a role in some – thiopentone anaesthetics for abdominal pain, barbiturates for the emotional crises typical of porphyria and for the hypertension, sometimes malignant, common in the family. I remember from my junior hospital doctor days that barbiturate night sedation was often routinely prescribed on hospital wards.

One woman (1.9.1) developed a porphyric crisis after a thiopentone anaesthetic in 1971, despite warning her gynaecologist and anaesthetist of the family history of similar events. Her story was corroborated by the consultant physician, Dr AC Hughes. In contrast, my index case, 1.6.5.3, and her second cousin, 1.8.3.7, had 31 admissions between them in the decade 1975–85 with no precipitating medication (Chapter 9), their attacks usually being premenstrual (Chapter 7).

## Chester porphyria today and tomorrow

Happily, very few members of the family are currently needing hospital admission for porphyric crises. This reduced incidence is difficult to explain, but has also been noted in South Africa.[19] As a result, our main duties are now counselling, education, and monitoring the long-term complications of porphyria. The main hope for the future is a reliable diagnostic test and an effective treatment or cure by gene therapy.

Kark wrote in 1955:

> ... *clinicians with an eye for color have long been fascinated with the lavender teeth of congenital porphyria, with the port wine urine excreted by some patients with intermittent porphyria and with the brilliant red fluorescence of the porphyrin pigments when they are exposed to ultraviolet light. Unfortunately the clinical course and management of disorders associated with gross porphyrinuria and porphyrinorrhea must still be painted in somewhat sombre hues.*[20]

The colourful story of the Dobson family and their complaint unfolds in the chapters to follow.

## References

1 Bennett A. *The Madness of King George III.* London: Faber & Faber, 1992.
2 Waldenström J. Neurological symptoms caused by so called acute porphyria. *Acta Psychiatrica et Neurologica* 1939; **14**: 375–9.
3 Qadiri MR, Youngs GR. Acute intermittent porphyria in Chester – a public health problem. *Gut* 1982; **24**: A487.
4 Qadiri MR, Church SE, McColl KEL, Moore MR, Youngs GR. Chester porphyria: a clinical study of a new form of acute porphyria. *British Medical Journal* 1986; **292**: 455–9.
5 Porteous CR. A case of porphyria complicated by pregnancies. *Journal of Obstetrics and Gynaecology* 1963; **70**: 311–4.
6 Shaper AG. Porphyria in Africa. *Central African Journal of Medicine* 1958; **4**: 411–20.
7 McColl KEL, Thompson GG, Moore MR, Goldberg A, *et al.* Chester porphyria: biochemical studies of a new form of acute porphyria. *Lancet* 1985; **ii**: 796–9.
8 Wang AL, Arredondo-Vega FX, Giampietro PF, Smith F, *et al.* Regional gene assignment of human porphobilinogen deaminase and esterase $A_4$ on chromosome 11q23→11qter. *Proceedings of the National Academy of Sciences of the USA* 1981; **78**: 5734–8.
9 Bissbort S, Hitzeroth HW, du Wentzel DP, Van den Berg CW, *et al.* Linkage between the variegate porphyria (VP) and the alpha-1-antitrypsin (PI) genes on human chromosome 14. *Human Genetics* 1988; **79**: 289–90.

10  Norton B, Lanyon WG, Moore MR, Porteous M, *et al.* Evidence for involvement of a second genetic locus on chromosome 11q in porphyrin metabolism. *Human Genetics* 1993; **91**: 576–8.

11  Norton B. *A genetic study of Chester porphyria.* MD thesis, University of Liverpool, 1993.

12  Church SE, McColl KE, Moore MR, Youngs GR. Hypertension and renal impairment as complications of acute porphyria. *Nephrology Dialysis Transplantation* 1992; **7**: 986–90.

13  Church SE. *The Chester porphyria.* MD thesis, University of Liverpool, 1986.

14  McColl KEL, Moore MR, Thompson GG, Goldberg A. Screening for latent acute intermittent porphyria: the value of measuring both leucocyte δ-aminolaevulinic acid synthase and erythrocyte uroporphyrinogen-1-synthase activities. *Journal of Medical Genetics* 1982; **19**: 271-6.

15  Diamond JM, Rotter JI. Observing the founder effect in human evolution. *Nature* 1987; **329**: 105–6.

16  Dean G. *The porphyrias, a story of inheritance and environment.* London: Pitman, 1963.

17  Haygarth J. Observations on the Bills of Mortality in Chester for the year 1772. In: Cassedy JH (ed). *Mortality in pre-industrial times – the contemporary verdict.* London: Gregg International Publishers, 1973.

18  Andrews J, Erdjument H, Nicholson DC. Hereditary coproporphyria: incidence in a large English family. *Journal of Medical Genetics* 1984; **21**: 341–9.

19  Hift R. *Variegate porphyria in South Africa.* International Association for the Study of the Liver, Cape Town, 1996.

20  Kark RM. Clinical aspects of the major porphyrinopathies. *Medical Clinics of North America* 1955; **39**: 11–30.

## Appendix

Letters expressing family members' lack of confidence in their medical advisers.

1 Letter from member of generation IV to Dr Bekerus (who left Chester in 1966), 3 October 1969:

*Dear Dr Bekerus*

*I am sorry to trouble you with my problems but I would be very grateful for your help.*

*My brother, ——, is to be admitted to Barrowmore Hospital on Tuesday to have his appendix removed. I think I mentioned when you were here that he has been having some stomach trouble. I have taken care to ensure that the Royal Infirmary, where he saw Mr ——, are aware of his blood condition but my mother is still rather anxious. I have assured her that so long as the hospital are aware that he has porphyria they will treat him correctly and now I am a little anxious myself. Do you think there will be any complications? I know that being in London you can have no bearing on what a Chester hospital does, but having been in the area at one time, do you think that the hospital officials will treat him in the correct manner? I do not for one moment doubt anyone's ability and possibly – indeed probably – his appendix does need to be removed, but having Uncle ——'s death still in our memory, you will, I'm sure, understand my concern. I would be grateful if you would give me a ring – please transfer the charges – just for a little reassurance.*

2 Letter from wife of member of generation III to Dr Bekerus, 25 May 1970:

*Dear Dr Bekerus*

*I hope you won't mind my writing to you, but Mr —— said just to let you know.*

*—— was taken into the City Hospital on the 21st with porphyria supposed just to be for 24 hrs. but he is still in and had a few tests as they don't really seem to know much about it.*

3 Letter from Dr Mary McBride, a Chester GP, to Dr DW Fielding, consultant paediatrician, Chester City Hospital, 31 May 1977:

*Dear David*

*You were kind enough, in 1972, to see Mrs ——, who suffers from porphyria, regarding her family. She is now in quite an anxious state which is justifiable due to the fact that her uncle died 13 weeks ago of it and her second cousin, aged 17, who was the uncle's son, also died last week of porphyria. She is very worried because when they go into hospital eg Wrexham, etc, nobody seems to know about the condition.*

*She would now like all five children tested to see which of them could be sufferers.*

*Chapter 2*

# Chester: a brief history of the city and the practice of medicine

GILES YOUNGS

## Roman Chester

Chester was the Roman *Deva*, and headquarters of the 20th Legion from the late 1st century. There were only three legionary fortresses in the British Isles, and no more than 30 in the whole Roman Empire. The name *Deva* is borrowed from the native name of the river, now the Dee, but more anciently *Deva*, Celtic for 'goddess' or 'holy one'.[1] The principal axes of the modern street pattern within the city are pure Roman, with four streets radiating from a central crossroads (Fig 6, Chapter 1). The foundations of many Roman buildings survive, including the biggest stone amphitheatre in Britain. The encircling medieval city walls, built in part upon the foundations of the Roman walls, are two miles in circumference and the most completely preserved in England.[2]

The fortress was built at the lowest bridgeable site on the River Dee, coincident with the upper limit of the tidal navigable river, and here the Romans built a port. In early medieval times (10th–14th century) Chester was one of the busiest ports in England and the main embarkation point for Ireland. The unique Rows, elevated walkways above street level, date from this time. Chester's maritime trade declined from the 16th century with the progressive silting of the River Dee.

## The practice of medicine in the Roman era

The earliest references to medical practice in Chester date from the Roman era, and reflect the fact that many of the doctors in the Roman Empire were Greek or Greek speakers.[3] Two altars dedicated by Greek doctors have been found in Chester, both in areas

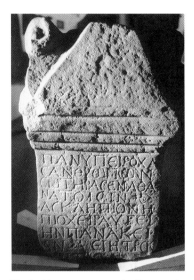

**Fig 1.** Altar stone set up by Doctor Antiochus recording the invocation to Asclepios of the gentle hands.

to the north of the legion's headquarters[4] – precisely where archaeologists believe the hospital would have been situated. The first reads:

*To the saviour gods – I Hermogenes the doctor set up this altar.*

The other (Fig 1) is more fulsome:

*The doctor Antiochus honours the all-surpassing saviours of men among the immortals, Asclepios of the gentle hands, Hygeia and Panacea.*

The latter inscription is reminiscent of the preamble to the Hippocratic Oath:

*I swear by Apollo, the Physician and Asclepios and Hygeia and Panacea and by all the gods and goddesses to keep according to my ability and my judgement the following oath ...,*[5]

– but it is probably a general invocation to the gods rather than the prelude to the Oath itself (V Nutton; personal communication). Both doctors, Hermogenes and Antiochus, were probably attached to the 20th Legion at the end of the 2nd century, practising in the same era as their illustrious colleague and fellow Greek speaker, Galen (died ca 216 AD) who, with Hippocrates (4th century BC), profoundly influenced western medicine for over a millennium. Voswinckel[6] and Rimington[7] both make a persuasive case that Hippocrates was the first to describe a case of acute porphyria in his *Epidemics Book III* which, in turn, like the Hippocratic Oath,[5,8] was the subject of a commentary by Galen.

## Medicine in Chester in the Middle Ages

Nothing is known of the practice of medicine in Chester through the 'dark ages' that followed the departure of the legions and the decline of Rome. More than a thousand years pass before the curtain begins to lift: in pre-Tudor 1475 there is a reference to the Company of Barber Surgeons, Wax and Tallow Chandlers[9] (an affiliation which doubtless present-day surgeons would find irksome).

Like many cities, Chester had trade guilds to encourage commerce, set wages, organise apprentices, and protect the livelihood of members by excluding outsiders, termed *forren* or 'foreigners'.[10] In the Middle Ages, members of the guild would follow the named trades after serving an apprenticeship for seven years. The Chester barber surgeons were prominent citizens, ranking with and exercising most of the functions of surgeons and physicians:

*They dressed wounds, drew teeth, bled their patients in more ways than one, made up ointments and pills, calculated to kill or cure, in all sorts of disorders as were to be found anywhere within our ancient walls.*[11]

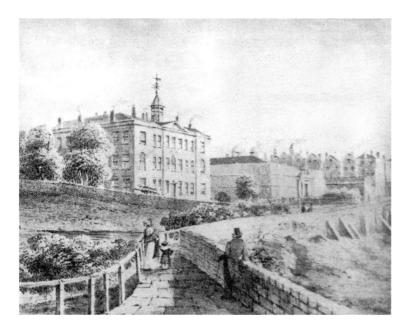

**Fig 2**. Chester Royal Infirmary, 1790: a view from the medieval city wall. On the other side of the wall from the infirmary is the site of the Roman port and the Roodee, the oldest racecourse still in use in the UK by about 100 years, some historians believing 1511 was the starting point and others favouring 1539. The course is unique in the anticlockwise gallop of the horses.[13]

The company's registers date from 1606 and record various disciplinary matters, for example:

*1651: fined Thomas Mortham two and six pence for wanting weight in his candles.*

*6 October 1658: Spent about putting down a forren barber in Hand-bridge … one shilling.*

Membership was strictly by inheritance in the male line so, in the course of time, persons not of that trade, but who were entitled to join by heritage, became members of the various Chester guilds. With so mixed a body, the special trades were no longer protected and many became extinct. By 1911, when Frank Simpson wrote his history of the company of Barber Surgeons, there was only one surviving member.[9]

Slowly – painfully slowly – 'rational' medicine ousted time-worn, irrational thought, and the mid-18th century age of enlightenment saw the foundation of many new hospitals.

## John Haygarth and the Chester Infirmary

Chester was among the first county towns to build an infirmary in 1755[12] (Fig 2). One of its earliest physicians (1767–98), John Haygarth (Fig 3), founded the Chester Small-Pox Society in 1778, which promulgated his doctrine of inoculation, isolation and sanitation, and greatly reduced the scourge of smallpox in Chester. He gained

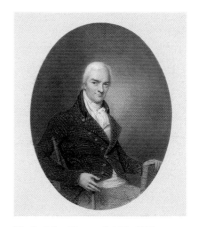

Fig 3. John Haygarth MD, FRS.

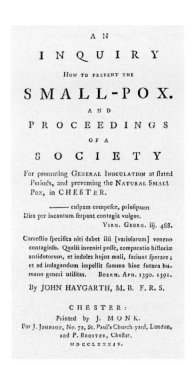

**Fig 4**. John Haygarth's Inquiry, 1784.

international renown by being the first to establish (in 1783) an isolation ward for infectious fevers, particularly smallpox.[14,15] His work was recognised by his election as a Fellow of the Royal Society in 1781, and he published his *Rules of Prevention* three years later[16] (Fig 4). Haygarth's visionary scheme for a nationwide and enforceable application of these Rules, published in 1793,[17] would have employed 500 inspectors directed by 50 physicians appointed by the King (George III) or the Royal College of Physicians, and paid for by the county rates. However, this scheme was not to be. By then, the nation had other priorities: war had broken out with France that year, and in 1798 Jenner's vaccination was introduced. Haygarth became a zealous advocate of Jenner's vaccination. In the second edition of his Inquiry (1801) he states that:

> *I had the good fortune successfully to convey the first Vaccine Contagion to the inhabitants of America through Professor Waterhouse.*

Waterhouse was Professor of Medicine at the new medical school at Cambridge (now Harvard) University in New England, which had awarded Haygarth an honorary MD in 1794.

## Chester's hospitals

In 1830, three years after Haygarth's death, we read that £3,250 was spent on alterations and additions to the *Chester Infirmary* (renamed the *Chester Royal Infirmary* in 1914) 'to care for patients suffering from hysteria, epilepsy and smallpox'. This foretells the events of a century later when subjects with Chester porphyria were often labelled incorrectly as having hysteria (Chapter 4, 6 and 11), and whose porphyric crises were sometimes complicated by epilepsy (Chapter 7). The hospital housed acute surgical patients until 1982, and was closed in 1996 (Fig 2, Chapter 1).

*Chester City Hospital* originated as the Chester Poor-Law Union Workhouse; it was built in 1877 and demolished in 1992. It housed the district's acute general medical beds for many decades until 1984.

The *Cheshire County Lunatic Asylum* (Fig 5; Fig 1, Chapter 11) was built in 1829 on the northern outskirts of Chester, and for more than 100 years received mentally ill patients from the whole county.[18] From 1921–50 it was called the County Mental Hospital (the title used in this book), from 1950–70, the Deva Hospital, and currently it is the West Cheshire Hospital. The 1829 Building has a fine façade and is listed as a building of architectural importance.

*Barrowmore Hospital* (Fig 2, Chapter 5), five miles east of Chester, founded in 1920, was the tuberculosis sanatorium for the

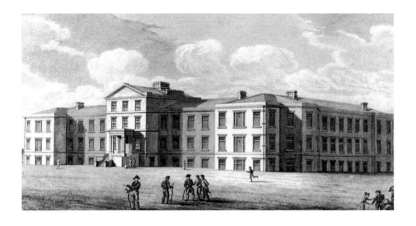

Fig 5. Cheshire County Lunatic Asylum (later County Mental Hospital), 1829.

district. It originally took cases of pulmonary tuberculosis in ex-servicemen, but subsequently accommodated non-urgent patients for most of the surgical subspecialties. It closed in 1982.

The *Countess of Chester Hospital*, so named after the official opening by Diana, Princess of Wales and Countess of Chester in 1984 (Figs 6 and 7), is adjacent to the West Cheshire Hospital. It is the district general hospital which has replaced the three defunct hospitals mentioned above.

*Clatterbridge Hospital* is a district general hospital 12 miles north-west of Chester serving the Wirral.

*Wrexham Maelor Hospital* is 12 miles south-west in Wrexham, Wales.

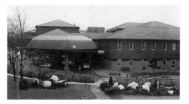

Fig 6. Countess of Chester Hospital, 1995 (opened in 1984).

## The changing scene

That a city of moderate size (80,000 inhabitants) had four hospitals, three of which provided surgical services, for most of the 20th century seems incongruous but reflects the history of health care provision in the UK. Between 1700 and 1825, 154 new 'voluntary' hospitals were founded.[19] This was the age of philanthropy when the care of the sick was no longer held to be primarily the duty of the Church. The Chester Royal Infirmary was maintained by charitable contributions from philanthropists and the local populace, supplemented by fees paid by patients who could afford them. The building of poor-law hospitals was a feature of Victorian times following the Poor-Law Amendment Act (1834) which set the framework of social welfare in the UK for the next 100 years. The resulting municipal hospitals were originally designed for the care of the destitute as well as for the sick poor. The consequent social stigma of admission to Chester City Hospital was very evident among the older citizens of Chester until the demolition of the hospital in 1992.

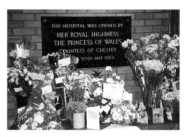

Fig 7. Plaque commemorating opening of the hospital in 1984. The photograph was taken in September 1997 a week after the death of Princess Diana. The flowers were placed by patients and staff.

Charles Wilson (later Lord Moran, personal physician to Winston Churchill, and President of the Royal College of Physicians from 1941–50) was a leading advocate of transforming poor-law infirmaries into modern hospitals.[20,21]

The fragmentation of medical care in Chester, finally corrected in 1996 by the unification of all the Chester hospitals on one site, had a deleterious effect on standards of medical practice. In particular, patients' case-notes and X-rays were often mislaid or in transit, and it was easy for hospital doctors to become professionally isolated from their colleagues in different disciplines. These factors undoubtedly delayed the recognition of the Chester porphyria, and impaired the medical management of porphyric illnesses. This disunion was mitigated by the foundation in 1883 of the Chester Medical Society. Reports of its proceedings were published in the *British Medical Journal* between 1885 and 1886. Its first President, Dr Edward Waters, had been President of the British Medical Association in 1866. The Society, now the Chester and North Wales Medical Society, continues to flourish.

# References

1 Thompson FH. *Deva – Roman Chester*. Chester: Grosvenor Museum, 1959.

2 Pevsner N, Hubbard E. *The buildings of England: Cheshire*. London: Penguin, 1971.

3 Nutton V. A Greek doctor at Chester. *Journal of the Chester Archaeological Society* 1968; **55**: 9–15.

4 Wright RP, Richmond IA. *Roman inscribed and sculptured stones in the Grosvenor Museum, Chester*. Chester: Chester and North Wales Archaeological Society, 1955.

5 Nutton V. What's in an oath? (College lecture) *Journal of the Royal College of Physicians of London* 1995; **29**: 518–24.

6 Voswinckel P. A constant source of surprises: acute porphyria. Two cases reported by Hippocrates and Sigmund Freud. *History of Psychiatry* 1990; **1**: 159–68.

7 Rimington C. Was Hippocrates the first to describe a case of acute porphyria? *International Journal of Biochemistry* 1993; **25**: 1351–2.

8 Rosenthal F. An ancient commentary on the Hippocratic Oath. *Bulletin of the History of Medicine* 1956; **30**: 52–87.

9 Simpson F. The City Guilds or Companies of Chester with special reference to Barber Surgeons. *Chester and North Wales Archaeological Society* 1911; NS **18**: 98–203.

10 Dobson J, Milnes Walker R. *Barbers and barber-surgeons of London*. Oxford: Blackwell Scientific Publications, 1979.

11 Elliott J. Chester. *British Medical Journal* 1912; **1**: 1311–9.

12 Boulton HE. The Chester Infirmary. *Journal of the Chester Archaeological Society* 1960; **47**: 9–19.

13 Bevan RM. *The Roodee – 450 years of racing in Chester*. Chester: Cheshire County Publishing, 1989.

14 Elliott J. A medical pioneer: John Haygarth of Chester. *British Medical Journal* 1913; **2**: 135–242.

15 Lobo FM. John Haygarth, smallpox and religious dissent in eighteenth-century England. In: Cummingham A, French R (eds). *The medical enlightenment of the eighteenth century*. Cambridge: Cambridge University Press, 1990.

16 Haygarth J. *An Inquiry How to Prevent the Small-Pox, and Proceedings of a Society for Promoting General Inoculation at Stated Periods, and Preventing the Natural Small-Pox, in Chester*. London: J Johnson, 1784.

17 Haygarth J. *A sketch of a Plan to Exterminate the Casual Small-Pox from Great Britain; and to introduce General Inoculation*. London: J Johnson, 1793.

18 Wall BA. *A world of its own: Chester's psychiatric hospitals, 1829–1976*. Chester: Cheshire Area Health Authority, 1977.

19 Cannon WG. Hospitals in the UK. In: Walton J, Barondess JA, Lock S (eds). *The Oxford medical companion*. Oxford: Oxford University Press, 1994: 376–83.

20 Wilson CM. The future of the poor-law infirmary. *Lancet* 1920; **ii**: 1287–90.

21 Wilson CM. Pay beds and the future of the voluntary hospitals. *British Medical Journal* 1928; **1**(Suppl): 85–7.

*Chapter 3*

# The Chester porphyria: notes on the social history of the Dobson family

ANDREW McDONAGH AND TERRY KAVANAGH

On first learning something about the Chester porphyria from reading the *British Medical Journal* paper of Qadiri *et al*[1] in 1986, the initial impression was that knowledge of the pedigree of the Chester kindred was already quite extensive. However, in addition to some minor inconsistencies in the facts then known about the Dobson family, there were further obvious aspects for future investigation. In particular:

- What was the line of inheritance of this porphyria which extended back before the 20th century?
- Could the genetic origin of the condition be linked with any other area of the world where porphyria is common?

This chapter concerns the first question and leads into the realms of genealogical research. Once embarked on this, a great deal of time was spent pursuing the family tree, with results that to date leave the original questions almost as tantalisingly open as at the outset. The search has, however, produced much of interest respecting the social history of the Dobson family, some of which may be instructive as background material to the main medical aspects of this book.

At the start of this genealogical study, one of us (AMcD) had no idea how difficult the proposed investigation would be, being quite unversed in the standard methods of the family historian, and learning the hard way about the use of official registration data for births, marriages and deaths, parish registers, census returns, monumental inscriptions, cemetery records, bastardy papers and the like. Due acknowledgement must also be made of the assistance of the Super-intendent Registrar for Chester and his staff, without whose help over several years the task would have been even more difficult.

## The start of the quest: Peter Dobson

*Generation I*

The initial objective was to confirm our information, previously gathered largely by word of mouth, on known members of the Dobson family. The kindred has been traced to a marriage in January 1888 at the Chester Register Office between Peter Dobson, a fisherman, and Sarah Ann Pay, daughter of a shoemaker from Wrexham. Peter Dobson, christened (10 June 1867) at the local parish church of St Mary on the Hill, Handbridge, Chester (Fig 1), was one of three illegitimate children of Ellen Dobson (herself christened at St Mary's 27 May 1839), whose surname he took. The *Chester Chronicle* of 8 June 1861 records that Ellen Dobson, prostitute, Handbridge, was charged at the city police court with throwing a lad, about nine years of age, into the canal on the previous evening. The identity of Peter Dobson's father is omitted from his birth certificate and remains obscure. The birth or christening records of more than 100 members of earlier generations of the Dobson family were then identified and tabulated as far back as the late 1780s. This information was obtained mainly from the parish registers of St Mary's Church, although the available registers for surrounding parishes and the Cheshire portion of the International Genealogical Index of the Church of Jesus Christ of the Latter Day Saints were also examined. Marriage records of these 18th and 19th

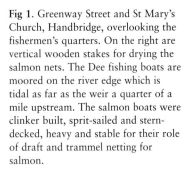

Fig 1. Greenway Street and St Mary's Church, Handbridge, overlooking the fishermen's quarters. On the right are vertical wooden stakes for drying the salmon nets. The Dee fishing boats are moored on the river edge which is tidal as far as the weir a quarter of a mile upstream. The salmon boats were clinker built, sprit-sailed and stern-decked, heavy and stable for their role of draft and trammel netting for salmon.

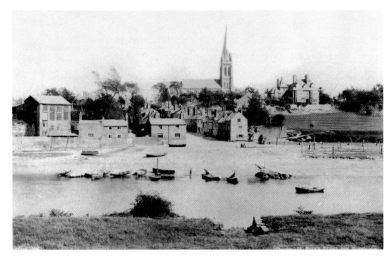

century Dobsons were sought out where possible, but information about their deaths remains limited. The results of this exercise are assembled in a large family tree (see endpapers). The Dobson family has been characterised by high fecundity and low rate of migration from Chester, both of which have facilitated the clinical and genealogical aspects of the study of Chester porphyria.

## Generation II

Peter Dobson had 14 children (generation II), of whom ten survived childhood (see Fig 3, Chapter 1). Acute hepatic porphyria is thought not to affect children, and there is certainly no evidence to the contrary in this kindred, so it was decided to confine our study to adult family members. The apparent preponderance of porphyria-positive individuals in generation II (at least 7 out of 10, and possibly all 10 siblings, see Chapters 1 and 6), and the high proportion of affected grandchildren (>60%) initially prompted the speculation that some unusual mechanism was involved in the inheritance of the porphyria gene – perhaps Peter Dobson's unknown father was a relative with the same genetic defect as his mother, and he was thus a homozygote. This is not wholly implausible because the probability of all 10 siblings inheriting an autosomal dominant trait from one heterozygote parent is 1:1,024. However, I (AMcD) consider the theory that one parent was homozygous because of a consanguineous union far from proven. Biological factors in addition to Mendelian laws may have been at work, for example, a porphyric embryo might have an enhanced chance of survival in the womb. We know that seven of the 10 siblings in generation II were porphyric, but the evidence that the remaining three were also porphyric is very circumstantial.

## Generation III

Nine of the 10 surviving children of this generation married and produced 43 grandchildren (generation III), of whom 38 survived childhood. These 38 were the issue of eight siblings, 35 of them porphyric. Sixteen of the 19 male grandchildren at risk of inheriting the porphyria gene did so – a distribution that would be expected to arise by chance with odds of 1:90.

## Generation IV

There are 106 great-grandchildren (generation IV). Of the 32 males and 26 females in generation IV known to be at risk of inheriting porphyria, 11 males and 14 females inherited it, indicating no evidence for an excess of porphyric members in this generation.

**Table 1.** Certified cause of death in senior members of the Dobson family.

| Name | Born or baptised | Died | Occupation | Relationship to Peter Dobson | Cause of death |
|---|---|---|---|---|---|
| George Dobson | 1776 | 1835 | Fisherman | Great-grandfather | Drowning* |
| William Dobson | 1806 | 1864 | Fisherman | Great-uncle | Typhus fever |
| Thomas Dobson | 1811 | 1885 | Fisherman | Grandfather | Natural decay |
| James Dobson | 1817 | 1875 | Fisherman | Great-uncle | Injuries received by accidentally falling a height of about 5 ft† |
| George Dobson | 1818 | 1854 | Slater & plasterer | Mother's cousin | Morbus cardis |
| Eliza Pay | 1835 | 1878 | Shoemaker's wife | Mother-in-law | Disease of heart & kidney |
| Samuel Dobson | 1823 | 1871 | Fisherman | Great-uncle | Drowning‡ |
| Robert Dobson | 1839 | 1858 | Not known | Mother's 2nd cousin | Decline |
| Samuel Dobson | 1845 | 1925 | Fisherman | Mother's brother | Senile decay. Acute bronchitis. Syncope |
| James Dobson | 1856 | 1939 | Retired river fisherman | 2nd cousin | Epithelioma of tongue |
| **Peter Dobson** | **1867** | **1932** | **Labourer§** | | **Carcinoma rectum** |
| Sarah Dobson (née Pay) | 1868 | 1921 | Fisherman's wife | Wife | Carcinoma kidney |
| Sarah Hand (née Dobson) | 1879 | 1921 | Labourer's wife | 2nd cousin | Intestinal paralysis |
| John Dobson | 1879 | 1922 | Gasworks stoker | 1st cousin | Endocarditis |
| Henry Dobson | 1886 | 1961 | Retired gas worker & River Dee fisherman | 1st cousin | Bronchopneumonia. Chronic bronchitis. Fractured neck femur |
| John Dobson | 1892 | 1916 | Munition worker | 2nd cousin | Morbus cardis. Cerebral haemorrhage. Syncope |

\* *Chester Chronicle* 13 March 1835
† The result of a fight (*Chester Chronicle* 29 May 1875)
‡ *Chester Courant* 8 April 1871
§ Previously fisherman

The information given in the table was obtained by a search of registers of death certificates of adults with the names of Dobson and Pay. Death certificates of numerous children were not perused. All the above are descendants of George Dobson (baptised 1776) and Elizabeth Mallard (died 1849), who married in Holy Trinity Church, Chester, in 1795.

## Death certificates

As will be discussed in Chapter 6 and elsewhere, erroneous or incomplete causes of death were frequently recorded on the death certificates of individuals dying from porphyria and its complications, even in quite recent years. Going back further in time, the certified causes of death become less specific, and probably less likely to reflect in any way now recognisable the manifestations of porphyria. Therefore, in addition, to the difficulty in obtaining the early death certificates, their usefulness to this study bears little relation to the effort involved in searching for them (a particular problem for individuals whose date of death is unknown and who might have left Chester).

In view of the large family size commonplace during the 19th century, it had been hoped to be able to detect a tendency for early deaths in some branch or branches of the family that might have been a marker for the porphyric phenotype as far back as the start of civil registration of deaths in 1837. Known certified causes of death for a small number of individuals predating generation II are given in Table 1, but unfortunately insufficient data are available from death certificates and burial records to allow this line of enquiry to be carried through at present.

## The trail of the porphyric phenotype

It remains unclear to what extent 20th century medicine has been responsible for provoking the acute clinical manifestations of porphyria. Before the advent of modern drugs, it may be that most cases of Chester porphyria remained latent, and detection in earlier generations may now be almost impossible. The current position is that the trail of the porphyric phenotype runs cold before the 1888 marriage of Peter Dobson and Sarah Ann Pay. It is not even certain that the gene for Chester porphyria was inherited through the Dobson rather than the Pay side of the family, although there is limited circumstantial evidence for porphyria in a different branch of the Dobson family (Chapter 6).

Still more important, if a genealogical link could be made, is the chance identification of porphyria, with investigations consistent with the biochemistry and genetic markers of Chester porphyria, in a spinster bearing the surname Dobson who moved to Chester from Warrington in the 1950s. Despite considerable effort, it has proved impossible to connect her with known ramifications of the Chester Dobsons. No deaths of members of the Pay family other than Sarah Ann and her mother, Eliza, have been traced.

## The fisher-folk of Chester

The occupation of Peter Dobson as a salmon fisherman on the River Dee (Fig 2) was mentioned in Chapter 1. The trade ran in families, and the lore of the river was passed from father to son.[3] Peter Dobson's great-grandfather, George (who married Elizabeth Mallard), his grandfather, Thomas, several great-uncles, uncles, and his brother Thomas were also fishermen (Table 1). His uncle, Samuel, was the most noted of these: among the exploits recorded in his

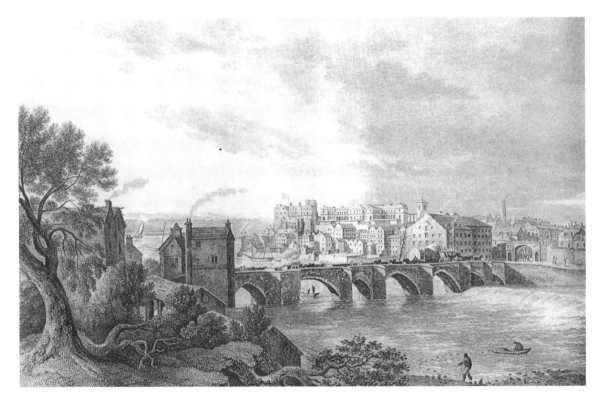

**Fig 2.** Chester from Handbridge showing use of draft net between old Dee Bridge and the weir.[2] Greenway Street is a quarter of a mile downstream. Salmon are caught by a draft or trammel net. The former is used on the upper stretches of the tidal River Dee opposite Greenway Street. A fisherman stays on the bank with the net end while a second rows the boat in a wide circle across the river, paying out the net until he returns to the bank a short distance downstream. Trammel netting is unique to the Dee estuary. The boat rows across the flow of the tide shooting the net which forms a vertical wall. The boat and net drift with the tide, the boat being manoeuvred by oar to keep the net across the tidal flow. In 1979 a full-time net fisherman could expect to catch 70–100 fish a year.[3]

obituary notice was a record haul of 80 salmon netted from a single tide in the 1860s when he was 17.

The social history of the fisher-folk has proved a fruitful and colourful source of research for one of us (TJK), a descendant of the Mallard family. Salmon fishing was a notable activity in Chester until the early years of the 20th century; it continues on a small scale today, with advertisements for netting licences appearing annually in the local press. In general, these fisher-folk were quite poor, living in proximity in a colony on the southern bank of the River Dee in the evocatively named Sty or Stye Lane (later named Greenway Street) area of the Handbridge district of Chester (Fig 1). Illegitimacy was common in this community. An example is to be found in the *Chester Chronicle* (2 September 1831):

> *William Totty, labourer was brought up by warrant, obtained by the assistant overseer of St Mary's Parish, to find sureties to abide orders in bastardy ... The female appeared in the person of Miss Hannah Dobson ... he [Totty] was committed to the House of Correction [the city gaol] until he could find sureties.*

Many of the families listed in the Dobson family tree had addresses in this street or in the immediate vicinity. A report in the *Chester*

*Chronicle* (12 October 1832), entitled 'Longevity in Chester', mentioned that:

> *in Greenway Street (vulgo, Sty Lane) in this City, there are at present living 81 persons who have attained the age of 60; twelve who are upwards of 80; and three who are near 90 years of age. There are not above 200 inhabitants in the whole street.*

So the conditions of deprivation and squalor were not an automatic recipe for early mortality.

In 1854, insanitary conditions in Stye Lane were a cause for concern to the Chester Board of Health, and a report in the *Chester Chronicle* (23 September) stated that:

> *In a nest of houses at the bottom of Stye Lane, not one was fit for human habitation, and in three families a most virulent diarrhoea, or cholerine, had broken out and in one family there had been four deaths. There was neither privy, convenience, ashpit, cesspool, coal shed, yard or water supply attached to any of these houses, and the cubic feet of space in the room, in which at least seven persons slept, was not equal to the required prison cell space for one person, in the model prisons of this country.*

The poverty consequent on large families and the variable profits of salmon fishing probably played their part in the frequent mention of Dobsons in the annals of justice. For example, the *Chester Chronicle* reported (7 December 1821) that George and Elizabeth Dobson were arraigned for assault after retrieving a fishing net from a bailiff, and (9 July 1853) that their son, Thomas (Peter Dobson's grandfather), was charged for illegally trammelling a net in the river and threatening to kill or do violent injury to Martha Nield if she dared to trammel her line before him.

Another report (12 January 1867) is worth quoting in full:

> *Elizabeth Dobson, a well-known fish hawker who lives in Stye Lane, and who appeared with a child in her arms (the poor little thing presenting a most sickly and emaciated appearance, having had one of its eyes knocked out and its left cheek burned or scalded), was charged with assaulting Sarah Holmes, who figured with a damaged 'phis' [face] and her eyes being in 'mourning'. Complainant said that on Thursday night defendant flew at her like a turkey cock, tore all the hair of her head and struck her over the face and other parts of the body several times. To give ocular demonstration of the injuries she had received, she bared her head in open court and it was proof positive that she had been transmogrified into a Chinese woman … The offence fully proved and a fine of 40 shillings and costs was inflicted, the option of payment being a month's imprisonment.*

Two of the family drowned (Table 1), one of them reported in the *Chester Chronicle* (13 March 1835) under the heading 'A case of real distress':

> *A poor fisherman named George Dobson, a native of Handbridge in this city, perished at sea under melancholy circumstances, in the severe gales in the month of January last, some miles outside the mouth of the river. A subscription has been set on foot for the relief of the widow and her orphan children, with a view to enabling her to purchase a boat, by which the eldest boy (whose intrepid conduct and providential escape are truly wonderful) will be enabled to support his mother and family. We recommend this case to the consideration of the humane and charitable.*

### The decline in the salmon fishing industry

Restrictive changes in the law governing salmon fishing were followed inevitably by declining fortunes for the Dobsons and their peers. By 1897, following a particularly bad salmon season, poverty was so extreme that 10 of every 12 wives amongst the 60–70 fishing families of Handbridge had pawned their wedding ring to obtain bread. In this era, the fishing colony was often seen as a 'lawless' place. The *Cheshire Observer* (13 July 1907) reported that:

> *In the City Police Court, a number of cross-summons taken out by members of the Greenway Street locality appeared on the list ... these were the result of 'supplementary quarrels' among members of the fishing fraternity ... with the consent of all parties the magistrates bound them over to keep the peace.*

With the continuing rundown of salmon fishing, Peter Dobson eventually gave up the struggle to make a living from the River Dee. His death was reported in the *Cheshire Observer* (10 December 1932):

> *Formerly a fisherman, the funeral procession of Mr Peter Dobson, 30 Greenway Street, Handbridge, in accordance with local custom, passed over both Dee bridges on the way to the cemetery on Monday. Mr Dobson who was 66 years of age, leaves a widow, five sons and five daughters, all married. Since 1914 he had been employed at Chester United Gasworks, but for nearly two years he had been away from work owing to illness.*

With the demise of river fishing on the Dee, the fishing colony was gradually dispersed, and many of the cottages in Greenway Street have been demolished. None of Peter Dobson's sons became a fisherman. The last reference to a Dobson (James) of Greenway Street being granted a netting licence is in 1936 (Clwyd Record Office, document DC/894). However, as recently as 1972, Thomas

44

Dobson, son of John Dobson and Sophia (née Hand), was still resident in Greenway Street according to the contemporary Kelly's directory.

Elizabeth Hughes (writing in a local amenity magazine *Friends of the Meadows*, Newsletter No. 32, February 1997) describes her early days as a resident in the street:

> *The fishermen in those days earned their entire livelihood by fishing the turbid waters of the Dee. We practically lived on the succulent Dee salmon and other varieties of fish such as flukes and slimy eels, which we called 'snigs'. Some of the fishermen cured the skins of eels and used them for remedial purposes. Our elderly neighbours wore them under scarves round their necks as poultices for sore throats, and they swore that they worked a treat.*

## References

1  Qadiri MR, Church SE, McColl KEL, Moore MR, Youngs GR. Chester porphyria: a clinical study of a new form of acute porphyria. *British Medical Journal* 1986; **292**: 455–9.
2  Ormerod G. *History of the County Palatine and City of Chester*, vol I. London: George Routlege, 1882.
3  Sweetnam J. *Salmon fishing on the River Dee*. Liverpool: Merseyside Maritime Museum, 1979.

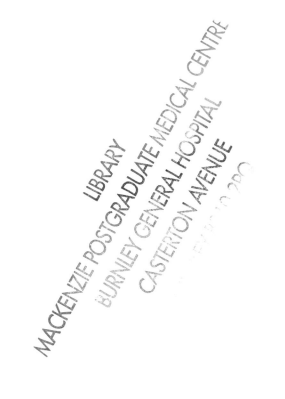

# Chapter 4

# A bizarre case of hypertension, uraemia, psychosis and paralysis: the first diagnosis of porphyria in the Chester kindred

COLIN PORTEOUS AND GILES YOUNGS

Subject 1.6.3 was the first member of our kindred to be diagnosed as having porphyria in 1954. We are fortunate in having some of her medical records. Her case will be described here in detail because she illustrates many of the fascinations of porphyria, including delayed diagnosis, suspicion of hysteria and long-term sequelae. Her malignant hypertension predated the advent of ganglion-blocking drugs. As related fully in Chapter 1, Dr AG Shaper, medical registrar to Dr RR Hughes at Clatterbridge Hospital, was the first to make the diagnosis of porphyria in 1954. Colin Porteous was obstetric registrar when he met the patient in 1958. Both published case reports.[1,2]

## Case history

### The first illness

1.6.3, age 23, had a healthy daughter of 14 months, and had previously been in good health until a caravan holiday in Rhyl, North Wales, in June 1954. She developed abdominal pains, and her mother-in-law noticed red urine in her chamber-pot. Her symptoms continued for some weeks, and she was admitted, because of abdominal pain and constipation, to Chester City Hospital on 28 August under the care of Dr AC Hughes, consultant physician. On examination, she had a tender abdomen, her blood pressure was 180/110 mmHg and blood urea 111 mg% (18 mmol/l). Her urine did not contain albumin or casts but was a 'funny browny red colour'. Within a few days she had an epileptic seizure, but her medication for this is not recorded. A nurse opined that 'there is nothing wrong with JB, only her bowels'.

*2 September 1954:* She became confused and disorientated. She was seen by Dr Dewi Jones, consultant psychiatrist, who diagnosed a 'depressive state with schizophrenic symptoms'. She was transferred to the County Mental Hospital under Section 20 of the Mental Health Act. She was found to be drowsy and restless with slurred speech, and complained bitterly of pains and paraesthesiae all over the body. Her blood pressure was 168/120 mmHg and she had bilateral papilloedema. Her tendon reflexes were equal and normal. Nurse's report: 'the patient is very poorly and appears delirious, complaining of pain in back, abdomen and legs. Very restless. Urine scanty and deep coloured'.

*4 September:* 'Drowsy this morning. Started on intravenous sodium sulphate' (a former treatment used for anuria and uraemia[3]).

*6 September:* 'Improved. Diagnosis type I nephritis. Urine: albumin trace (10 mg%)'.

*10 September:* Blood pressure 180/120 mmHg and blood urea 138 mg% (23 mmol/l). Seen by Dr GA Kiloh, consultant physician. Diagnosis: chronic nephritis; 'prognosis hopeless'.

She improved rapidly over the next three weeks in the County Mental Hospital, with resolution of the uraemia and papilloedema, although the hypertension persisted. Unfortunately, during this period she received 12 grains (720 mg) of barbiturate drugs. By 5 October she had developed a complete flaccid paralysis of both arms and legs, with blood pressure of 150/115 mmHg. A lumbar puncture on the 10th day of paralysis showed a normal cerebrospinal fluid, but it was followed by five severe epileptiform convulsions in one hour which were treated with intramuscular Luminal (phenobarbitone sodium) 2 grains (120 mg).

An opinion was requested of Dr RR Hughes, visiting consultant neurologist from the Royal Southern Hospital, Liverpool, and the patient was transferred to one of his beds at Clatterbridge Hospital. Dr Langsten, senior psychiatric registrar at the County Mental Hospital, records in a subsequent letter (to Dr Hughes' registrar, Dr AG Shaper):

*Whilst she was in the hospital many of the nursing staff believed she was suffering from a form of hysteria, and one found it difficult to convince them otherwise. This, I think, was due to the sensation in her paralysed limbs remaining intact and she was subjected to many cramps and paraesthesiae and because of her paralysis being unable to ease herself by movements, this necessitated calling out to the nurses for more attention than superficially appeared necessary.*

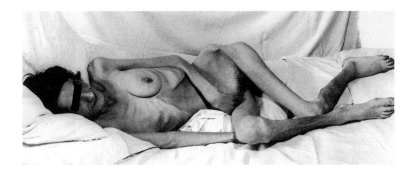

**Fig 1**. Subject 1.6.3 during her first illness in 1954–55, showing severe emaciation (weight 25 kg) and flexion contractures.

*15 October*: Clatterbridge Hospital (clerking and most of subsequent entries by Dr Shaper). 'Further major seizure. Emaciated. Complete flaccid paralysis of arms and legs. Cannot speak. Wasting of muscles and absent reflexes. No loss of sensation to light, touch or vibration. No papilloedema. Blood pressure 120/68 mmHg. Blood urea 66 mg% (11 mmol/l).

*3 November*: Seen by orthopaedic surgeon because of flexion contracture of both hips and knees. Galvanic and faradic stimulation prescribed. Weight 4 st (25 kg) (Fig 1).

*30 November*: Blood pressure 160/130 mmHg. 'She appears to be going into uraemic hypertensive state, similar to the one she experienced before'. She developed sudden blindness and became confused and restless. The optic fundi were pale with the arterioles in spasm and she had marked neck rigidity. She was treated with prostigmine and paraldehyde. Blood urea 34 mg% (6 mmol/l), serum sodium 340 mg% (148 mmol/l). The laboratory reported: 'This urine contains porphyrins which fluoresce with ultraviolet light and gives a positive test for porphobilinogen and porphyrinogens.'

*4 December*: 'Vastly improved. No further abdominal pain. Blood pressure 175/135 mmHg. Blood urea 84 mg% (14 mmol/l). Weight 4 st 4¼ lb (27 kg). Urine: no casts, faint trace of protein.'

*25 December*: 'Restless, confused, shouting. Screaming with fright, then major epileptic seizure. Blood pressure 230/165 mmHg.' Papilloedema was again noted with exudates, haemorrhages and a perimacular 'star'.

*10 January 1955*: 'Electroencephalogram grossly abnormal. The record indicates a state of generalised brain damage. It is impossible to say whether this abnormality is due to a direct action of porphyrins or whether it is due to hypertension or impaired renal function.'

*7 February:* Intravenous urogram normal. Papilloedema increased.

*23 February*: 'Movement very good indeed. Still has marked weakness of extensors of wrists and fingers. Blood pressure 190/150 mmHg. Increased number of exudates in right eye with papilloedema. Blood urea 36 mg% (6 mmol/l). Urine: trace of protein only.'

*3 March*: 'Looks wonderfully well. Can even feed herself. Has taken her first few steps. Weight 4 st 9½ lb (30 kg).'

*25 March*: Started on Serpasil (reserpine) qid, with fall of her blood pressure to normal over the next two weeks.

*12 April*: 'Tendon reflexes present. Left optic fundus normal, exudates improving on right. To remain on Serpasil 2 tablets qid.'

*16 June*: Discharged home from Clatterbridge Hospital with continuing physiotherapy arranged for foot drop. Weight 5 st 10 lb (36 kg).

*13 July*: Outpatient visit. 'Suffered daily headaches. Blood pressure 110/85 mmHg.'

*12 October*: Outpatient visit. 'Well except for some headache and back pain. Weight 6 st (38 kg). Blood pressure 150/105 mmHg. Tendon reflexes all diminished. Muscle power commensurate with wasting. Sensation normal to all modalities. Optic fundi normal.'

*11 January 1956*: 'Improved. Blood pressure 150/100 mmHg. Weight 6 st 5 lb (40 kg). Electroencephalogram still abnormal but much improved.'

*22 May*: 'Very well. Blood pressure 140/95 mmHg. Urine still contains porphobilinogen. Blood urea 42 mg% (7 mmol/l).'

*10 October*: 'Very well. Blood pressure 150/80 mmHg. Blood urea 65 mg% (11 mmol/l).'

In 1957 she was well, and able to care for her home and her family without assistance. In March 1958 she was tried on Inversine (mecamylamine hydrochloride) for painful cramps in the limbs. It reduced her blood pressure from 170/110 mmHg to 150/80 mmHg, but her general practitioner (GP) was advised to prescribe it only for intermittent use for cramps, which it seemed to help. On 20 September 1958 she reported that she was 12 weeks pregnant.

### Second pregnancy*

Six years after the birth of her first baby, the patient, then aged 29 years, reported again in the 17th week of her second pregnancy. She weighed 98 lb (44½ kg), her blood pressure was 150/100 mmHg, and urinalysis was normal except for a trace of uroporphyrin. The haemoglobin level was only 62% and so she was treated with oral iron. Except for a mild hypertension, the patient remained well and was admitted for rest and observation at the 34th week of gestation. Her blood pressure was then 140/90 mmHg, haemoglobin 52%, and blood non-protein nitrogen 27 mg/100 ml. The urine was strongly positive for porphobilinogen and darkened on standing.

On admission, the patient was treated by rest, a diet restricted in salt and fluids, and a transfusion of two pints of packed blood cells. After

*The account of her second and third pregnancies is extracted from the report by Porteous.[2]

the latter, the haemoglobin level rose to 78%. When she had been treated for two weeks her blood pressure was 180/120 mmHg, and the urine contained free haemoglobin and 4 g/l of albumin. Labour was therefore induced by artificial rupture of the membranes. During labour, injections of morphine, pethidine and histidine (200 mg in 5 ml) were given. A live male infant weighing 3 lb 15 oz was delivered after an easy labour lasting 12½ hours, but he survived for only 24 hours. Post-mortem examination revealed that the cause of death was atelectasis.

In the puerperium, the patient was given histidine injections (200 mg in 5 ml) intramuscularly twice daily for three days and then daily for a week. On the fourth day, the blood pressure was 180/115 mmHg, blood non-protein nitrogen 85 mg/100 ml, and haemoglobin 76%; six weeks later, these values were 135/85 mmHg, 35 mg/100 ml and 80%, respectively. The urine was then free from albumin, but contained porphobilinogen and uroporphyrin. The patient was advised against pregnancy and given advice about contraception.

## Third pregnancy

The contraceptive advice was not followed, and the patient reported again in July 1961 when she was 12 weeks pregnant. Termination of pregnancy was suggested, but was opposed by the patient.

She weighed 96 lb (44 kg), her blood pressure was 130/80 mmHg, and her haemoglobin 59%. Treatment with oral haematinics was instituted but, despite this, the haemoglobin level was only 45% at the 32nd week of gestation and she was admitted.

On admission, her weight was 110 lb (50 kg), her blood pressure 140/90 mmHg, and the urine contained albumin. The haemoglobin rose to 76% following slow transfusion with two pints of packed blood cells and a course of intravenous iron. The blood pressure rose to 190/110 mmHg and the blood non-protein nitrogen was 38 mg/12200 ml. Treatment with oral guanethidine sulphate 20 mg daily, and histidine (200 mg in 5 ml) by intramuscular injection twice daily was given, with good effect.

By the 37th week of pregnancy the haemoglobin level had fallen to 58%, and a further two pints of packed cells were transfused. Following this, the patient went into labour spontaneously; 4½ hours later, when the cervix was fully dilated, the fetal heart rate began to slow. A low forceps delivery under local anaesthesia was undertaken, and a live female infant weighing 5 lb 6 oz was delivered. The woman's blood pressure at this time was only 130/90 mmHg.

On the fourth day of the puerperium, histidine was discontinued but was recommended the following day because her blood pressure increased to 210/150 mmHg; guanethidine sulphate was also continued. The patient's condition improved rapidly, and in the second week of the puerperium abdominal sterilisation was carried out under general anaesthesia. Examination of the liver and kidneys during this operation

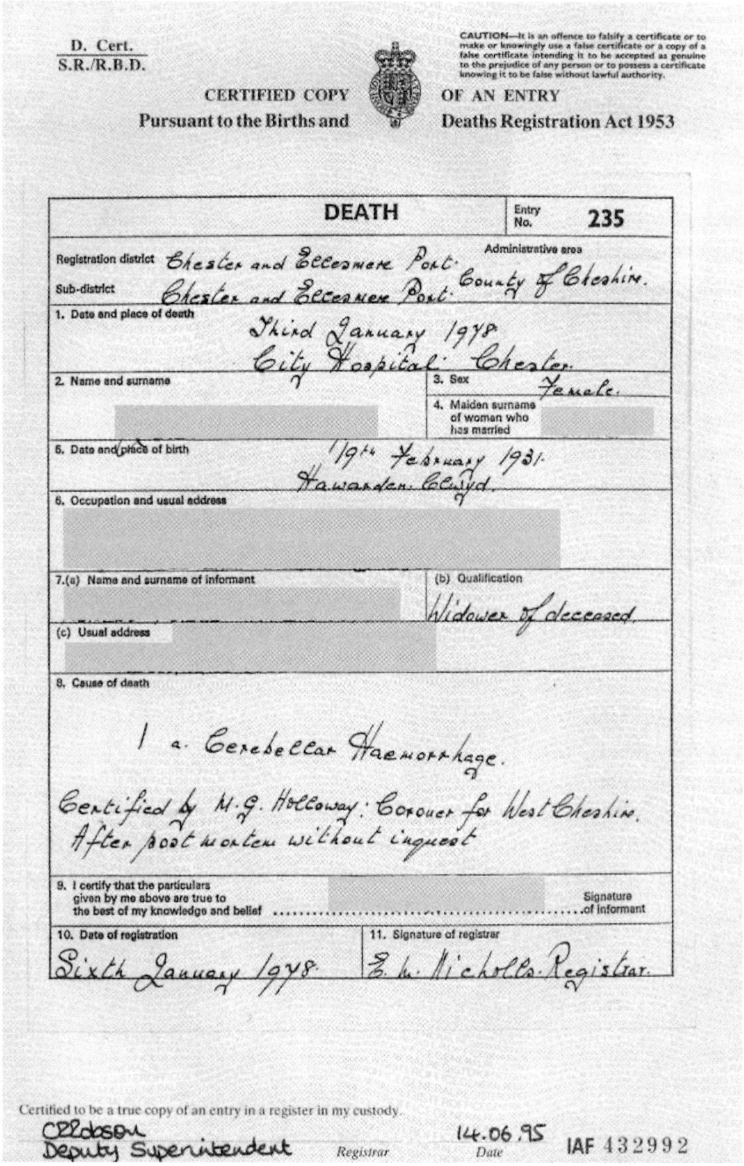

Fig 2. Death certificate of subject
1.6.3.

revealed no abnormality. Six weeks later, the blood pressure was
130/100 mmHg and she was well, despite not having any treatment.
The baby, who had been artificially fed since birth, was thriving.

*27 January 1967*: She was referred to Dr Kiloh by her GP, Dr RH
McClure.* The patient complained of headaches and her blood pressure was 240/130 mmHg (previously 185/100 mmHg, 170/110 mmHg
and 220/110 mmHg in 1962, 1964 and 1966, respectively). In the
outpatient clinic, her blood pressure was 250/140 mmHg and optic
fundi showed grade I hypertensive changes. Routine urine testing was

negative for protein. Blood urea was 44 mg% (7 mmol/l) and average urea clearance 21% of normal. ECG, chest radiograph and intravenous urogram were all normal. Her blood pressure was observed, and finally she was admitted for treatment.

*September 1967*: Admitted to Chester City Hospital. Blood pressure 255/150 mmHg. Optic fundi showed grade III hypertensive changes. Blood urea 77 mg% (12 mmol/l) and 105 mg% (17 mmol/l). She was treated with Ismelin (guanethidine) and her blood pressure fell to 150/80 mmHg.

*September 1968*: Blood pressure was 200/100 mmHg recumbent and 170/80 mmHg erect. Blood urea was 50 mg% (8 mmol/l) and serum sodium 140 mmol/l. Treatment continued with guanethidine 50 mg daily.

*October 1969*: Blood pressure 210/100 mmHg supine, 170/90 mmHg erect. Her optic fundi showed grade II hypertensive changes.

It appears that she was lost to hospital follow-up thereafter, but Dr McClure referred her to the ophthalmic clinic in 1974 because of a tic, and stated that she was still on guanethidine 50 mg daily. No ocular abnormality was seen.

*January 1978* (age 46): She was admitted to the Chester City Hospital after sudden headache and loss of consciousness. Dr McClure noted that she had been on guanethidine 62.5 mg for 10–12 years. Blood pressure was 240/180 mmHg. A clinical diagnosis of subarachnoid haemorrhage was made, and she died one hour later. Post-mortem examination by Dr TDS Holliday showed haemorrhage into the right lobe of the cerebellum with enlargement of the heart, particularly the left ventricle. The kidneys were both considerably shrunken with granular subcapsular surfaces. The histology is described in Chapter 8. Her death certificate (Fig 2) merely records the cerebellar haemorrhage.

## Discussion

The sad story of our subject illustrates many of the tribulations that can be suffered by victims of the acute hepatic porphyrias. She was suspected of hysteria by nurses in two hospitals at a time when she was paralysed to the extent of not being able to speak or adjust her own position in bed. Waldenström[4] quotes a GP who advised that:

*when somebody dies from hysteria in this province she usually suffers from acute porphyria.*

We too, both nurses and doctors, in Chester find it difficult to judge the true need for opiate analgesia in porphyric patients with abdominal and muscle pain. The marked weight loss in subject 1.6.3 is reminiscent of the autobiographical report, recorded by Dean,[5] by a doctor with porphyria variegata whose weight fell from 230–110 lb during a porphyric illness.

The question of who made the diagnosis of porphyria in subject 1.6.3 is of historical interest only, but nevertheless it is of some fascination (see Chapter 1). Only the previous year (1953) two cousins had died of what we believe to have been porphyric illnesses:

> *1.5.3*: died age 30 years in the Chester City Hospital of pneumonia, paralysis and peripheral neuritis.

> *1.2.8*: died age 18 years of left ventricular failure and malignant hypertension 12 days after discharge from the County Mental Hospital (Table 3, Chapter 6).

In addition, three cousins (brothers of 1.2.8) had died of paralysis in the 1940s.

The subject of this chapter, 1.6.3, was the first member of the pedigree to be diagnosed as having porphyria. Had porphyria not been diagnosed, she would almost certainly have received more barbiturates and probably died. The porphyric illness of her brother, 1.6.5, in 1958 and the death of her cousin, 1.9.3, from paralysis in the same year may not have been recognised as being due to porphyria. Family knowledge of the diagnosis obviously assisted their medical advisers to stumble upon the explanation for subsequent victims' symptoms. Thus, subject 1.5.2 was probably saved a third dose of barbiturates (Chapter 6) when the family history was disclosed, but forewarning did not prevent subject 1.9.5 receiving a barbiturate anaesthetic with disastrous consequences (Chapter 6).

*Pregnancy and porphyria*

The association between pregnancy and porphyric crises is well reported. Neilson and Neilson[6] described two deaths from porphyria complicating pregnancy, and their review of the literature revealed that 95% of 40 subjects with porphyria became worse in pregnancy. Goldberg's group[7] found that 54% of 50 women had an attack in pregnancy or the puerperium, and they described[8] a pregnancy complicated by severe neuropathy similar to our own case. These authors reported that the first attack in females often occurs during pregnancy, and that attacks in pregnancy are more common in previously symptomatic, as opposed to latent, porphyrics. They advised patients not to consider pregnancy until they have been free of symptomatic attacks for 18 months, but rarely considered termination of pregnancy in patients with acute porphyria – and then only in very severe attacks in early pregnancy. Kauppinen and Mustajoki's experience in Finland[9] is less worrying. They described 176 deliveries in 76 women with either acute intermittent or variegate porphyria, most of whom were not known to have porphyria at the time. Porphyric symptoms occurred in only 14 pregnancies (in 12 women, of whom nine were primigravida), half of whom went on to develop an acute porphyric attack post-partum. Four of the 12 women had further symptomless pregnancies.

Pregnancy-related symptoms do not feature strongly in members of our pedigree, although a formal retrospective or prospective study has not been undertaken. Subject 1.9.1 died from a pregnancy-related accidental haemorrhage in 1963. She is of unknown porphyric status. Her sister, 1.9.3, died age 22 in 1958 in the 16th week of her first pregnancy after developing abdominal pain, hypertension and pharyngeal paralysis. Urine was positive for porphobilinogen, and her death certificate, which recorded acute respiratory failure and porphyria, was the first death certificate in the kindred to report porphyria.

## Steroid hormones and porphyria

Further evidence that steroid hormones are porphyrogenic is provided by the fact that many attacks in women occur premenstrually.[10,11] This was particularly striking in our two subjects, 1.6.5.3 and 1.8.3.3, whose 31 hospital admissions due to porphyric crises were often premenstrual (Chapter 7).

An explanation for the effect of steroid hormones is found by a consideration of the enzyme changes in the normal menstrual cycle. Porphobilinogen deaminase levels in erythrocytes decrease sharply between the 17th and 24th days of a normal menstrual cycle,[12] and serial leukocyte alanine-synthase activity shows a peak prior to menstruation.[11] For these reasons, most authors advise that the contraceptive pill is unsafe in porphyria,[8,13] but Kauppinen and Mustajoki's[9] experience allows room for leniency. Forty-four of the 95 women with porphyria in their series had used sex hormone preparations, and fewer than 5% experienced an acute attack during therapy, so a causal relationship was uncertain. They therefore allow the use of the contraceptive pill under supervision, but advise strict avoidance in symptomatic subjects.

## Administration of histidine

We presume that histidine was prescribed in the second and third pregnancies of subject 1.6.3 following the evidence that this agent may alleviate experimentally-produced porphyria in the chick

(EL Talman; personal communication, quoted in Ref 6). This indication for histidine was never recognised in the *British Pharmacopoeia*, and only sceptical reference was made to its use in the treatment of peptic ulcer and arteriosclerosis obliterans in *Martindale's Extra Pharmacopoeia* (24th edition).[14] We have not discovered any contemporary use of histidine in obstetric practice or for hypertension.

*Long-term complications of porphyria*

The hitherto under-recognised long-term complications of porphyria manifest in subject 1.6.3, hypertension and chronic renal failure, are discussed in Chapter 8.

### References

1 Shaper AG. Porphyria in Africa. *Central African Journal of Medicine* 1958; **4**: 411–20.

2 Porteous CR. A case of porphyria complicated by pregnancies. *Journal of Obstetrics and Gynaecology of the British Commonwealth* 1963; **70**: 311–4.

3 *Martindale's Extra Pharmacopoeia*, 23rd edn. London: Pharmaceutical Press, 1952.

4 Waldenström J. The porphyrias as inborn errors of metabolism. *American Journal of Medicine* 1957; **22**: 758–73.

5 Dean G. *The porphyrias, a story of inheritance and environment*, 2nd edn. London: Pitman Medical, 1971.

6 Neilson DR, Neilson RP. Porphyria complicated by pregnancy. *The Western Journal of Surgery, Obstetrics and Gynecology* 1958; **66**: 133–49.

7 Brodie MJ, Moore MR, Thompson GG, Goldberg A. Pregnancy and the acute porphyrias. *British Journal of Obstetrics and Gynaecology* 1977; **84**: 726–31.

8 Moore MR, McColl KEL, Rimington C, Goldberg A. *Disorders of porphyrin metabolism*. New York: Plenum, 1987.

9 Kauppinen R, Mustajoki P. Prognosis of acute porphyria: occurrence of acute attacks, precipitating factors, and associated diseases. *Medicine* 1992; **71**: 1–13.

10 Perlroth MG, Marver HS, Tschudy DP. Oral contraceptive agents and the management of acute intermittent porphyria. *Journal of the American Medical Association* 1965; **194**: 1037–42.

11 McColl KEL, Wallace AM, Moore MR, Thompson GG, Goldberg A. Alterations in haem biosynthesis during the human menstrual cycle: studies with normal subjects and patients with latent and active acute intermittent porphyria. *Clinical Science* 1982; **62**: 183–91.

12  Batlle AMC, Wider de Xifra EA, Stella AM. A simple method for measuring erythrocyte porphobilinogenase and its use in the diagnosis of acute intermittent porphyria. *International Journal of Biochemistry* 1978; **9**: 871–5.

13  *British National Formulary*. London: British Medical Association and the Royal Pharmaceutical Society, 1995.

14  *Martindale's Extra Pharmacopoeia*, 24th edn. London: Pharmaceutical Press, 1958.

.

# Chapter 5

# Complications after nasal polypectomy: a family tree is constructed

ZORKA BEKERUS (*WITH NOTES BY GILES YOUNGS*)

This chapter has been adapted from a manuscript written by Dr Zorka Bekerus (Fig 1a) in 1965 but never published, although in that year she presented a paper to the Anaesthetic Section of the Royal Society of Medicine (London), for which she received the Registrar's Prize (Fig 1b), and to the Liverpool Society of Anaesthetists.

Zorka Bekerus qualified in medicine in Belgrade, Yugoslavia, in 1955 and was anaesthetic registrar to the Chester Hospitals in 1963–65. She administered the anaesthetic to case 1.1.5 at Barrowmore Hospital (Fig 2) and, having made the diagnosis of porphyria, decided to study the family in depth. Many family members remember her visiting them at home and collecting repeated urine samples. She subsequently informed the subjects of their porphyric status by letter (see example, Fig 4, Chapter 1). After Bekerus left Chester in about 1966 she received anxious enquiries from members (Appendix, Chapter 1).

Bekerus subsequently settled in New York, and it took nine years to trace her. In 1989, she kindly sent me the manuscript reproduced in this chapter,* the family tree, and case histories – which amazingly she had kept. Family memories of causes of death, and Bekerus' recordings of blood pressure, renal function and urine testing for porphobilinogen by the Watson–Schwartz method[1] proved invaluable and added to the data we published in 1985[2] and 1986.[3] Bekerus records that only two members were previously known to have

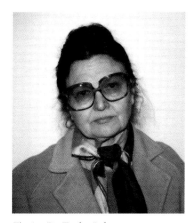

Fig 1a. Dr Zorka Bekerus.

---

*The extracts are verbatim except for minor editorial changes and the addition of the modern family notation.

59

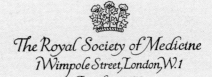

The Royal Society of Medicine
1 Wimpole Street, London, W.1
Langham 2070

SECRETARY: R. T. HEWITT, O.B.E., M.A

18 February 1965

Dear Dr. Bekerus,

    Section of Anaesthetics  -  Registrar's Prize.

      I am writing to you with pleasure to tell you formally that the Council of the Society, at a meeting earlier this week, approved the recommendation from the Council of the Section of Anaesthetics that the Registrar's Prize for 1965 be awarded to you. There is, as you know, an award of £50, and I enclose herewith a cheque for that amount.

      I should like to offer you Council's congratulations, together with my own, on this occasion.

          Yours sincerely,

          R. T. Hewitt

Dr. Zorka Bekerus,
9 Tavistock Road,
Wallasey,
Cheshire.

**Fig 1b.** Dr Bekerus received the Registrar's Prize from the Royal Society of Medicine, 1965.

suffered from porphyria, but in fact three cousins of her index case had been diagnosed by this time (Chapter 1).

Porteous' case history of 1.6.3 published in 1963[4] is not mentioned by Bekerus or included in her references, perhaps because it was written from a different hospital (Clatterbridge) and escaped her notice.

## Case history, subject 1.1.5

A man of 35 years was admitted for nasal polypectomy in 1963. He was premedicated with morphine 10 mg and atropine 0.6 mg, and anaesthesia was induced with 350 mg thiopentone and 50 mg suxamethonium. Anaesthesia was maintained with nitrous oxide, halothane and oxygen. During induction, it was noted that the facial muscles were unduly lax. Fifteen minutes after induction spontaneous breathing was inadequate and the patient was cyanosed. Controlled ventilation by hand was therefore started and continued for the 30-min duration of the operation. Post-operatively, spontaneous respiration was still inadequate and assisted manual ventilation was continued for another 30 min. On return to the ward the patient complained of severe headache and later abdominal pain. A diagnosis of appendicitis was considered, but a

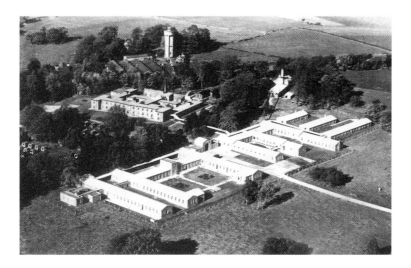

Fig 2. Barrowmore Hospital in the 1950s. The building in the midground was built during the Second World War after the original hospital was destroyed by a land mine in November 1940. Among trees on the extreme left can be seen the wooden chalets in which the tuberculous patients slept.

further anaesthetic was thought inadvisable and surgery was postponed. The next day red urine was observed and the diagnosis of porphyria occurred to me.

The patient had a long history of headaches, abdominal pain, constipation and profuse sweating, with backache and leg pains following exertion. He had recurrent pustules on his face, usually in the spring, which led to scarring (Fig 3).

I kept the patient in hospital for investigation. He was confused and complained of headache, weakness, aches and pains. He had sustained hypertension of 180/130 mmHg, blood urea of 110 mg (18 mmol/l), and urine positive for porphobilinogen by the Watson–Schwartz test. An intravenous pyelogram showed poor concentration of dye but no obstruction. The following investigations were normal: haemoglobin, erythrocyte sedimentation rate, blood glucose, serum electrolytes, liver function tests, Wassermann reaction, bone marrow, creatinine clearance, Rogitine (phentolamine mesylate) test for phaeochromocytoma, radiographs of chest and bones. He was discharged from hospital on the 10th day but his urine was still red.

[Dr Bekerus does not record whether the patient received any night sedation before the operation. This was common practice in the 1960s, and barbiturates were frequently prescribed.]

*Investigation of the family of subject 1.1.5*

I decided to interview other members of the family and constructed a family tree (Fig 4). I traced 132 members, of whom 24 were dead. Only two members were previously known to have suffered from porphyria. I have seen and physically examined 100 members. Urine has been tested for porphyria two or more times in 91 members. By previous history, I have diagnosed 30 members to have porphyria: 12 are dead, 10 have urine positive for porphobilinogen by the modified Watson–Schwartz

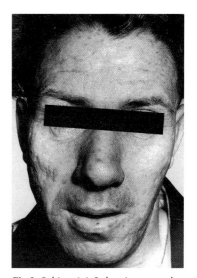

Fig 3. Subject 1.1.5 showing scarred face.

**Fig 4.** Family tree showing generations I–IV (Bekerus, 1965):

□ = male;

○ = female;

■, ● = cases diagnosed by history *and* urine examination;

◪, ◑ = cases diagnosed by history *or* urine examination;

† = dead;

⊟ = not investigated (refused investigation, inaccessible or dead);

V = had thiopentone anaesthesia.

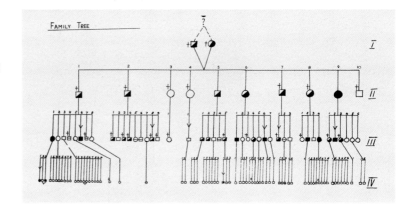

Table 1. Excretion products in the acute hepatic porphyrias (Bekerus, 1965).

| Porphyria hepatica | Inheritance | Skin changes | Barbiturate sensitive | Excretion | |
|---|---|---|---|---|---|
| | | | | Urine | Faeces |
| South African (porphyria variegata) | Mendelian dominant | Cutaneous fragility. Sores & scars leave pigmentation (often) | Yes | *Acute*: increased porphyrins, PBG, ALA | *Acute*: increased copro- & protoporphyrins |
| | | | | *Remission*: normal | *Remission*: increased copro- & protoporphyrins |
| Chester | Mendelian dominant | Fragility. Prone to infection, scars | Yes | *Acute*: increased porphyrins, PBG, ALA | *Acute*: increased copro- & protoporphyrins |
| | | | | *Remission*: increased porphyrins, PBG | *Remission*: increased copro- & protoporphyrins |
| Swedish (acute intermittent porphyria) | Mendelian dominant | None | Yes | *Acute*: increased porphyrins, PBG, ALA | *Acute*: slightly increased porphyrins |
| | | | | *Remission*: increased porphyrins, PBG, ALA | *Remission*: normal |

ALA = delta-aminolaevulinic acid

PBG = porphobilinogen

method, six have negative urine (two over the age of 60), and two refused urine examination (one of whom had a mental illness and paralysis possibly produced by barbiturates). The youngest subject with positive urine was 15 years old and the oldest 50. Taking the first three generations (excluding the fourth [generation] whose members are all below the age of 20), approximately 60% of this family are affected by porphyria.

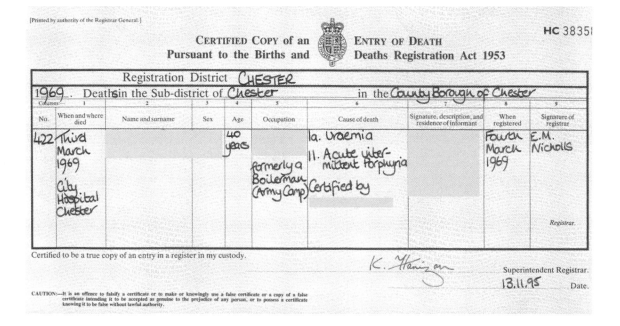

[Printed by authority of the Registrar General.]

**CERTIFIED COPY of an**
**Pursuant to the Births and**

**ENTRY OF DEATH**
**Deaths Registration Act 1953**

HC 3835

Registration District _CHESTER_

1969. Deaths in the Sub-district of _Chester_ in the _County Borough of Chester_

| No. | When and where died | Name and surname | Sex | Age | Occupation | Cause of death | Signature, description, and residence of informant | When registered | Signature of registrar |
|---|---|---|---|---|---|---|---|---|---|
| 422 | Third March 1969 City Hospital Chester | | | 40 years | formerly a Boilerman (Army Camp) | 1a. Uraemia 11. Acute inter-mittent Porphyria Certified by | | Fourth March 1969 | E.M. Nicholls Registrar. |

Certified to be a true copy of an entry in a register in my custody.

_K. Hanigan_

Superintendent Registrar.

13.11.95  Date.

CAUTION:—It is an offence to falsify a certificate or to make or knowingly use a false certificate or a copy of a false certificate intending it to be accepted as genuine to the prejudice of any person, or to possess a certificate knowing it to be false without lawful authority.

Six subjects with urine positive for porphobilinogen provided urine and stool samples for quantitative spectroscopic tests (performed at Alder Hey Children's Hospital, Liverpool). Porphobilinogen was present in the urine both in the acute attack and in remission. Similarly, copro- and protoporphyrins were present in both phases. As shown in Table 1, the excretion products seem to be intermediate between acute intermittent porphyria and variegate porphyria.

I was struck by the fact that members of the family are symptomatic only between puberty and the climacteric, and that many male members were relatively infertile – indeed, eight males died in middle age unmarried. Ten members had received thiopentone anaesthesia, but it seemed not to harm prepubertal or post-climacteric subjects.

Differential diagnoses include hysteria, psychoneurosis, acute abdomen, polyneuritis, polymyositis, and renal colic. The principal danger to a patient with porphyria is to misdiagnose the problem and treat with barbiturates – this led to some members of the family being admitted to the mental hospital. In remission or in latent porphyrics I found certain features of practical value in diagnosis: sallow complexion, emotional instability, fragile skin which easily became infected, headaches, fatigue, constipation and colic. The males were single or married late, but the women were very fertile.

Subject 1.1.5 died in 1969 age 40 years, only six years after meeting Bekerus. His death certificate records uraemia, hypertension and acute intermittent porphyria (Fig 5). The medical records have been destroyed.

Fig 5. Death certificate of subject 1.1.5.

63

## Discussion of Bekerus' findings

Bekerus' study is valuable for many reasons, and the biographical and medical details of the family she recorded 30 years ago have proved both fascinating and valuable. I salute both her industry and her ability to give me her manuscript 25 years later. Family members remember her with affection. She was the first to note the higher than expected proportion of the family afflicted by porphyria, identifying 30 positive members (61%) in the first three generations of 49 subjects (Mendelian theory would predict 31%). Admittedly, many of her cases were diagnosed by history only, which can have its dangers (C Rimington; personal communication 1969, quoted in Ref 5). She was also the first to suggest that the porphyrin excretion products in urine and stools in our subjects are intermediate between acute intermittent and variegate porphyria.

Bekerus notes that her subject had recurrent pustules on the face which led to scarring (Fig 3); on questioning, she found that some other family members were prone to sunburn and boils. She postulates (Table 1) that our family demonstrates the dermatological features of porphyria variegata. Neither of the porphyria-positive sisters of 1.1.5 (1.1.1, 1.1.6) had skin problems, and 1.1.6 remembers her brother's skin ailment being labelled acne. I have not come across any other members of the pedigree with skin fragility or scarring as seen in porphyria variegata or porphyria cutanea tarda.

One other cousin (1.6.5) developed a porphyric crisis after nasal polypectomy (Chapter 6), his brother (1.6.1) has nasal polyps, and two members of the next generation (1.1.1.1, 1.9.1.2) have asthma and nasal polyps. The prevalence of asthma, atopy and nasal polyps in the kindred is discussed in Chapter 10.

Bekerus' assertion of relative male infertility is not fully substantiated by a study of the up-to-date family tree (see endpapers). Of the 10 children of Peter and Sarah Dobson, the four porphyric daughters and three porphyric sons produced 16 and 19 children, respectively. The eight porphyric granddaughters and 16 porphyric grandsons produced 30 and 27 children, respectively. The discrepancy in the fecundity of the male and female grandchildren is largely accounted for by the fact that none of the six sons of subject 1.2 married, four of them dying of porphyria under the age of 30 years (Table 3, Chapter 6).

*Postscript (GRY)*

After preparing this manuscript Dr Bekerus provided me with further details of the preamble to her first encounter with porphyria.

Because of post-operative abdominal pain, subject 1.1.5 was transferred from Barrowmore Hospital to the Chester Royal Infirmary.

*The next day as I (ZB) was walking through the corridor of the Royal Infirmary, a new and young lady house officer informed me that she had just premedicated a patient for acute appendicitis with morphine and atropine for surgery in an hour. When I went to check the patient, I was surprised in recognising Mr ____. Remembering the problems with anaesthesia the day before, I asked that surgery be postponed. The next day the house officer told me 'your patient Mr ____ is passing urine as red as your blouse' (and I was wearing a very red blouse!). I then remembered a lecture by the late Professor John Dundee delivered to the Liverpool Postgraduate Course in Anaesthetics early in 1963. He told us that acute porphyria is the only absolute contraindication for the use of thiopentone. I subsequently read his recently published article on the subject.[6] The course was organised by the Professor of Anaesthesia, Cecil Gray, and it was he who subsequently encouraged me to present my story to the Royal Society of Medicine.*

Zorka Bekerus adds:

*I remember quite vividly Mr ____ as a patient, and later his entire family. He was a very humble and gentle man, and the entire family was always gracious and cooperative even if they did not participate in the testing. I was very sorry that I could not have helped them more than advising them of the condition existing in the family.*

# References

1 Watson CJ, Schwartz S. A simple test for urinary porphobilinogen. *Proceedings of the Society for Experimental Biology and Medicine (NY)* 1941; **47**: 393–4.
2 McColl KEL, Thompson GG, Moore MR, Goldberg A, *et al*. Chester porphyria: biochemical studies of a new form of acute porphyria. *Lancet* 1985; **ii**: 796–9.
3 Qadiri MR, Church SE, McColl KEL, Moore MR, Youngs GR. Chester porphyria: a clinical study of a new form of acute porphyria. *British Medical Journal* 1986; **292**: 455–9.
4 Porteous CR. A case of porphyria complicated by pregnancies. *Journal of Obstetrics and Gynaecology of the British Commonwealth* 1963; **70**: 311–4.
5 Dean G. *The porphyrias, a story of inheritance and environment*, 2nd edn. London: Pitman, 1971.
6 Dundee JW, McCleery WNC, McLoughlin G. The hazard of thiopental anaesthesia in porphyria. *Anesthesia and Analgesia – Current Researches* 1962; **41**: 567–74.

*Part 2*

# Dobson's complaint mystifies and eludes the Chester doctors

*Chapter 6*

# Mortality in the kindred: a story of premature deaths and incomplete or incorrect death certificates

MOHAMMAD QADIRI AND GILES YOUNGS

Peter Dobson, a salmon fisherman on the River Dee, was born illegitimate in 1867 and died in 1932 of rectal carcinoma. He is remembered to have had asthma. His wife, Sarah, died age 53 in 1921 of renal carcinoma. We have been unable to trace the death certificates of any of her family except that of her mother, Eliza Pay, who died age 43 years in the County Mental Hospital of disease of the heart and kidneys (Chapter 11). Peter's mother, born in 1839, was one of at least 34 cousins, and we have traced the death certificates of some of the numerous members of Peter's family (Table 1, Chapter 3). His second cousin, John Dobson, who was also a member of the fishing community in Greenway Street, died age 24 in 1916, the death certificate recording morbus cardis, cerebral haemorrhage and syncope. John's sister Sarah, wife of a general labourer, died age 41 in 1921 at the Chester Royal Infirmary of intestinal paralysis. The certified cause of death in both cases is reminiscent of many recorded in porphyric subjects later in this chapter. Their brother, William, was convicted of murdering their aunt in 1927.

## Generation II (10 siblings): clues to possible porphyria markers

Peter and Sarah Dobson had 10 children who reached adulthood, born between 1890 and 1911, and who died between 1938 and 1982. The mean age of death was 54 years (range 32–83 years). Urine assayed for porphobilinogen was positive in the only two

**Table 1.** Causes of death in generation II (10 siblings).

| Family notation | BMJ notation[1] | Sex | Age at death (years) | Death certificate | Other previous morbidity | Notes |
|---|---|---|---|---|---|---|
| *Subjects with porphyria* | | | | | | |
| 1.1 | II.6 | M | 48 | Lobar pneumonia | Paralysis (ZB) | Obligatory carrier |
| 1.2 | II.5 | M | 62 | Obstructive airways disease. Hypertension | | Obligatory carrier |
| 1.4 | II.1 | F | 59 | Pneumonia. Cerebral thrombosis | | Obligatory carrier |
| 1.5 | II.9 | M | 83 | Pulmonary embolus. Uraemia. Chronic urinary retention. Pernicious anaemia | | Obligatory carrier |
| 1.6 | II.4 | F | 81 | Bronchopneumonia. Senile dementia | | Obligatory carrier. Urine PBG (1982) |
| 1.8 | II.2 | F | 31 | Lobar pneumonia | | Obligatory carrier |
| 1.9 | II.8 | F | 59 | CVA. Acute intermittent porphyria | | Obligatory carrier. Urine PBG (1963) |
| *Porphyric state unknown* | | | | | | |
| 1.3 | II.10 | F | 48 | Uraemia. Hypertension. Atheroma of aorta | | Only child died young |
| 1.7 | II.7 | M | 35 | Influenzal pneumonia | Confusional insanity. Headaches | 3 offspring (1 negative, 1 not tested, 1 died appendicitis) |
| 1.10 | II.3 | M | 38 | Coronary thrombosis | Paralysis of arms (ZB) | No children |

BMJ = British Medical Journal
CVA = cerebrovascular accident
Urine PBG = urine positive for porphobilinogen
(ZB) = word of mouth information from Dr Zorka Bekerus in 1963

tested (1.6 in 1980, 1.9 in 1963). Death certificates are available for all 10 siblings, on one of which acute intermittent porphyria was mentioned (1.9) (Table 1).

*1.9*: wife of a labourer, born in 1908 and died in 1967. She had a history of agitation, and abdominal and back pain. In 1949, she complained of these symptoms during a gynaecological hospital admission and was prescribed amylobarbitone sodium, 3 grains (180 mg) as night sedation. Her death certificate records cerebrovascular accident (CVA) and acute intermittent porphyria. Three of her six children inherited porphyria, which caused death in two (1.9.3, 1.9.5).

Seven siblings, including the two sisters with positive urine tests, are obligatory carriers of porphyria because their children are

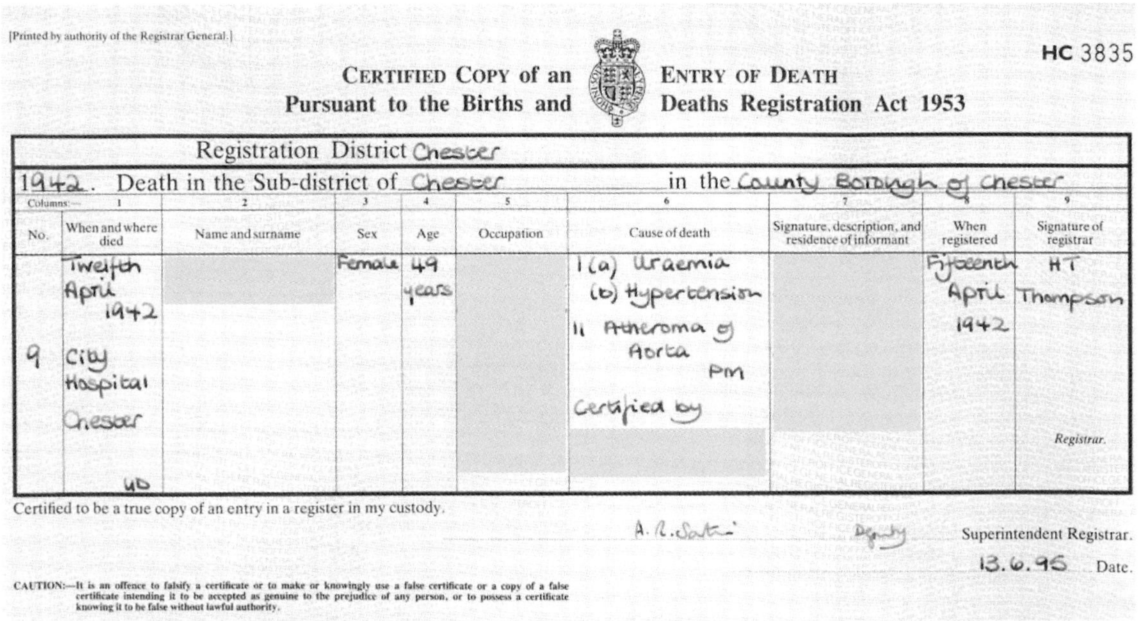
[Printed by authority of the Registrar General.]

HC 3835

CERTIFIED COPY of an ENTRY OF DEATH
Pursuant to the Births and Deaths Registration Act 1953

Registration District Chester

1942. Death in the Sub-district of Chester in the County Borough of Chester

| No. | 1 When and where died | 2 Name and surname | 3 Sex | 4 Age | 5 Occupation | 6 Cause of death | 7 Signature, description, and residence of informant | 8 When registered | 9 Signature of registrar |
|---|---|---|---|---|---|---|---|---|---|
| 9 | Twelfth April 1942 City Hospital Chester UD | | Female | 49 years | | I (a) Uraemia (b) Hypertension II Atheroma of Aorta PM Certified by | | Fifteenth April 1942 | HT Thompson Registrar. |

Certified to be a true copy of an entry in a register in my custody.

A. R. Sat... Deputy Superintendent Registrar.

13.6.95 Date.

CAUTION:—It is an offence to falsify a certificate or to make or knowingly use a false certificate or a copy of a false certificate intending it to be accepted as genuine to the prejudice of any person, or to possess a certificate knowing it to be false without lawful authority.

**Fig 1.** Death certificate of subject 1.3.

porphyric. The porphyria status of the remaining three siblings is not known, but they had complaints frequently suffered by their porphyric nephews and nieces but not by their porphyria-negative peers. They died age 48, 31 and 37, and two of them had no surviving issue.

*1.3*: wife of a general labourer, born in 1893 and died in 1942. Her death certificate records uraemia, hypertension and atheroma of the aorta (Fig 1). Her only child died in infancy.

*1.7*: a labourer, born in 1904 and died in 1940 in the County Mental Hospital, having been transferred there three years before with confusional insanity and severe pains in the head. The case-notes are incomplete and record neither his medication nor any other specific porphyria symptoms such as paralysis. His death certificate records influenzal pneumonia.

We wondered if this was a porphyric death, but have no supporting evidence from study of his offspring: two of his children (1.7.2, 1.7.3) have negative tests, and the third, 1.7.1, died in Australia in 1956 age 31 years from 'appendicitis', which Bekerus surmised may have been porphyric abdominal pain but she gives no evidence for this. The three children of 1.7.1 live in Australia; two have been tested for porphyria, with negative results.

*1.10*: builder's labourer, born in 1911 and died in 1949. His death certificate records coronary thrombosis, but Bekerus was told he had paralysis of his arms. He had no issue.

Thus, of the three siblings of unknown porphyria status, the two brothers died in their 30s, one after a psychiatric illness and one with a family memory of paralysis; their sister died age 49 of uraemia and hypertension. Psychiatric illness, paralysis, uraemia and hypertension are common afflictions in the porphyric grandchildren but not in their porphyria-negative siblings (as will be seen later). If these three diagnoses are markers of porphyria, it raises the intriguing possibility that all 10 siblings had porphyria (see Chapters 1 and 3).

Paralysis is not mentioned on any of the siblings' death certificates, but subject 1.1 was said to have died of 'creeping paralysis' according to his daughter, 1.1.6. Hypertension is recorded on two (1.2, 1.3) of the 10 death certificates. In addition, 1.4, 1.5 and 1.6 are known from hospital records to have been hypertensive. Uraemia is recorded on two certificates (1.3, 1.5), but may have been due to chronic urine retention in 1.5. Two siblings are known to have had admissions to the County Mental Hospital, 1.7 (see above) and 1.8, who had a history of stomach pains and admissions to the County Mental Hospital with delirium before dying aged 31 years of pneumonia. All her three children (1.8.1–3) had considerable porphyria morbidity (Table 3 and Chapter 7)

## Generation III (38 grandchildren): the cause of their poor life expectancy is not at first recognised

Peter and Sarah Dobson had 43 grandchildren, 38 of whom survived childhood. These 38 were the issue of eight siblings (1.1–2, 1.4–9), seven of whom were porphyria-positive. The status of the remaining sibling, 1.7, is unknown (as noted in the case history above). Twenty-one of the 38 grandchildren died aged between 16 and 72 years (average age of death 41 years). The porphyria status of the 38 grandchildren, 24 of whom we believe to be porphyric, is summarised in Table 2.

Table 2. Summary of porphyria status of living and dead grandchildren (generation III).

| Grandchildren | Porphyria-positive | | | Porphyria-negative | | |
| | Biochemical | Obligatory | History only | Biochemical | Unknown status | Total |
| --- | --- | --- | --- | --- | --- | --- |
| Living | 8 | 0 | 0 | 8 | 1 | 17 |
| Deceased | 10 | 2 | 4 | 1 | 4 | 21 |
| All subjects | 18 | 2 | 4 | 9 | 5 | 38 |

It is noteworthy that only one of the nine biochemically-negative subjects (1.1.3) has died (in 1993 age 72 years from acute cardio-respiratory failure and pneumonia), but that 10 of the 18 biochemically-positive subjects have died. In addition, both obligatory porphyrics have died. There is strong circumstantial evidence that four brothers (1.2.1, 1.2.3, 1.2.4, 1.2.8) died of unrecognised porphyria at the age of 29, 21, 16 and 18 years, respectively (their case histories are recorded later in the chapter).

Summarising mortality in generation III:

- Twenty-one of the 38 grandchildren have died, including 16 whom we believe to be porphyric, while all but one of the biochemically-negative members are still living.
- The excess deaths in the porphyric grandchildren (16 out of 24) occurred over a period of 47 years.
- Ten of those deaths occurred before the age of 50, some recognised as being due to porphyria and others not.

## Deaths in the grandchildren probably due to unrecognised porphyria

We have the death certificates of 17 of the 21 deceased grandchildren, including those of 15 of the 16 porphyric grandchildren who have died (Table 3). Hospital case-notes are available for a few but, in general, these and general practitioners' (GPs) records were destroyed five years after death. Family memory has been useful, especially regarding paralysis. Further information has come from family histories routinely recorded by house physicians and surgeons in relatives' hospital case-notes over the years (our thanks to all of them for their diligence).

Four brothers died at an early age between 1941 and 1953 from what we believe to have been unrecognised porphyria. None of the four had children. Their father (1.2) died age 62 in 1953, his death certificate recording obstructive airways disease and hypertension. There is no record or family memory of him having symptoms of porphyria. He is an obligatory porphyric because one surviving son (1.2.6) had a positive blood test (reduced porphobilinogen deaminase) in 1989, although no porphyria symptoms. Bekerus' notes on this family are recorded in Chapter 1.

*1.2.1*: died age 29 in 1946 in the Chester City Hospital. His death certificate records uraemia, acute nephritis and mental deficiency. Bekerus records 'rheumatic first, paralysed hands, mentally affected'.

*1.2.3*: general labourer, died age 21 in 1943 in Chester Royal Infirmary. His death certificate records myotonia atrophica (Fig 2). Bekerus was told 'paralysed legs, bowel problem'.

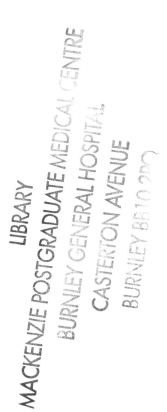

**Table 3.** Details of generation III (38 grandchildren) who have died.

| Family notation | BMJ notation[1] | Sex | Age at death (years) | Death certificate | Morbidity | Notes |
|---|---|---|---|---|---|---|
| *Subjects with porphyria* | | | | | | |
| 1.1.1 | III.25 | F | 63 | Cerebellar haemorrhage. Hypertension | | Urine PBG (1963). Obligatory carrier |
| 1.1.5 | III.21 | M | 40 | Uraemia. Hypertension. Acute intermittent porphyria | Porphyric crisis after nasal polypectomy | Urine PBG (1963). ZB index case* |
| 1.2.1 | III.15 | M | 29 | Uraemia. Nephritis. Mental deficiency | Paralysed hands (ZB) | These 4 brothers died betwen 1941 & 1953. We feel there is strong circumstantial evidence that these were porphyria-related deaths. Another brother (1.2.6) was biochemically positive. |
| 1.2.3 | III.13 | M | 21 | Myotonia atrophica | Paralysed legs (ZB) | |
| 1.2.4 | III.12 | M | 16 | Pneumonia. Operation appendicitis | Paralysed legs (ZB) | |
| 1.2.8 | III.14 | M | 18 | Left ventricular failure. Malignant hypertension | Died 12 days after leaving County Mental Hospital | |
| 1.5.1 | III.35 | M | 60 | Unobtainable | Porphyric crisis after barbiturates. Psychiatric illness | Urine PBG (1963) |
| 1.5.2 | III.39 | M | 67 | Ischaemic heart disease. Aspiration pneumonitis. Bleeding gastric ulcer | Porphyric crisis after barbiturates. Psychiatric illness | Urine PGB (1964) |
| 1.5.3 | III.36 | M | 30 | Pneumonia. Paralysis. Peripheral neuritis | Psychiatric illness treated with barbiturates | Obligatory carrier |
| 1.5.5 | III.38 | M | 51 | Acute heart failure. Atherosclerosis. Bronchitis | Psychiatric history. Clinical meningitis but no evidence at necropsy | Obligatory carrier |
| 1.6.3 | III.7 | F | 46 | Cerebellar haemorrhage | Malignant hypertension. Uraemia. Paralysis. Psychosis† | Urine PBG (1954). Obligatory carrier |
| 1.6.4 | III.8 | F | 58 | Bronchopneumonia. Chronic obstructive airways disease | | Blood PBGD (1983). Obligatory carrier |
| 1.6.5 | III.10 | M | 37 | Cerebral haemorrhage. Malignant hypertension. Porphyria | Abdominal pain. Porphyric crisis after nasal polypectomy | Urine PBG (1958). Obligatory carrier |
| 1.8.3 | III.3 | F | 47 | Renal failure. Acute intermittent porphyria | Abdominal pain. Red urine | Urine PBG (1963). Obligatory carrier |
| 1.9.2 | III.34 | M | 55 | Intracerebral haemorrhage. Hypertension. Acute intermittent porphyria. Chronic renal failure | Peripheral neuropathy. Psychiatric illness | Urine PBG (1963). Blood PBGD (1983) |
| 1.9.3 | III.30 | F | 22 | Acute respiratory failure. Porphyria | Abdominal pain. Red urine | Urine PBG (1958) |

**Table 3** *continued*

| Family notation | BMJ notation[1] | Sex | Age at death (years) | Death certificate | Morbidity | Notes |
|---|---|---|---|---|---|---|
| *Porphyric state unknown* | | | | | | |
| 1.2.2 | III.16 | M | 62 | Not available | | Urine PBG negative (1963) |
| 1.2.5 | III.18 | F | 58 | Not available | | Not tested |
| 1.7.1 | III.26 | M | 31 | Not available | Died after operation for 'appendicitis' in Australia | Not tested |
| 1.9.1 | III.32 | F | 31 | Accidental haemorrhage (childbirth) | | Not tested |
| *Porphyria-negative subject* | | | | | | |
| 1.1.3 | III.24 | M | 72 | Acute cardiorespiratory failure. Pneumonia | | Normal PBGD (1983) |

\* see Chapter 5
† see Chapter 6

Blood PBGD = reduced porphobilinogen deaminase
*BMJ = British Medical Journal*
Urine PBG = urine positive for porphobilinogen
(ZB) = word of mouth information from Dr Zorka Bekerus in 1963

*1.2.4*: died age 16 in 1941 in the Chester Royal Infirmary. His death certificate records pneumonia and operation (appendicitis). Bekerus was told he had paralysed legs and pneumonia.

*1.2.8*: died age 18 in 1953 in the Chester City Hospital. His death certificate records left ventricular failure and malignant hypertension. A year earlier he had an operation for appendicitis. He became paralysed and confused, and had a voluntary admission to the County Mental Hospital. He was discharged and died 12 days later. We have seen the hospital case-sheet, but the details are scanty and the medication unrecorded.

Two brothers from a different family, who were cousins of the four brothers described above, have a similar story.

*1.5*: their father, died age 83 in 1980 in the County Mental Hospital. His death certificate recorded pulmonary embolus, uraemia, chronic urine retention and pernicious anaemia. He presented in 1963 with a six-year history of abdominal pain, but routine investigations were negative. In 1967, he developed monoplegia and hypertension but had a normal blood urea. He has obligatory porphyria because one son (1.5.2) is biochemically positive, but porphyria was not recognised in the two other sons described below.

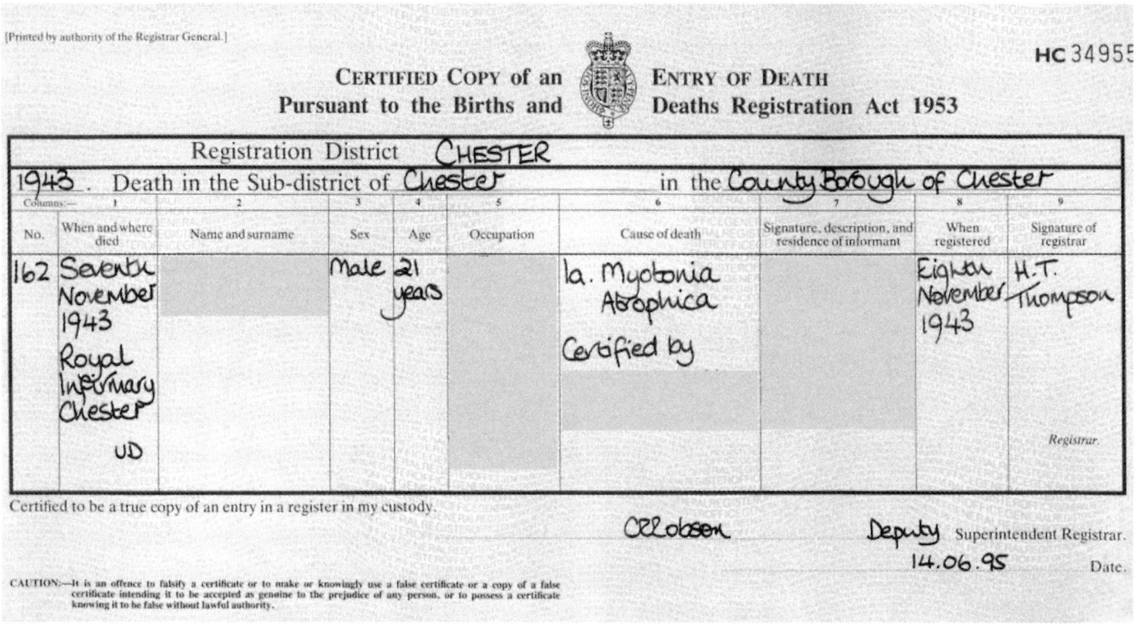

**Fig 2.** Death certificate of subject 1.2.3.

*1.5.3*: driver/salesman of an ice cream van, died age 30 in 1953 in Chester City Hospital after being admitted with abdominal pain suspected to be due to peptic ulcer. His death certificate records hypostatic pneumonia, paralysis and peripheral neuritis (Fig 3). Bekerus was told he had an odd personality and used to drink vinegar. She records that he was treated with barbiturates. All his three children are biochemically positive for porphyria.

*1.5.5*: unemployed taxi driver, died age 50 in 1982 in Chester City Hospital. His death certificate records acute heart failure, atherosclerosis and bronchitis. He became depressed after marital separation, and was admitted to the County Mental Hospital after being found at home lying on the floor. He had been taking triazolam, diazepam and co-proxamol. He weighed 6 st 8 lbs (42 kg), but had been described as obese in the orthopaedic clinic five years earlier. During admission, he complained of difficulty swallowing, weakness in the limbs, hallucinations, severe anxiety, and had three major epileptic seizures. He heard voices and developed bizarre behaviour (eg he licked urine off the floor). Inpatient drugs included amitriptyline, clomipramine, nomifensine, diazepam, chlorpromazine and trifluoperazine.

Three months later, still in hospital, he became comatose, with tachycardia, pyrexia, neck stiffness, papilloedema and generalised increase in muscle tone. He was transferred to the Chester City Hospital with a diagnosis of either meningitis or CVA. Blood pressure, serum sodium and urea were normal, and papilloedema was again noted. He died two days after transfer without a clinical diagnosis. Post-mortem examination showed no intracranial abnormality. His medical advisers were

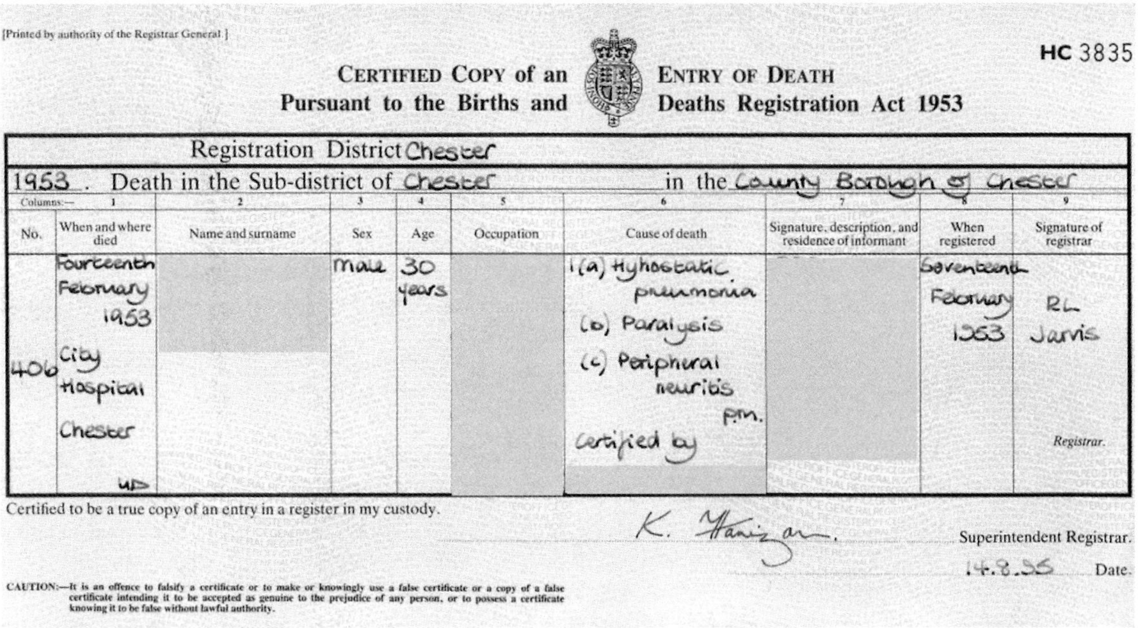

[Printed by authority of the Registrar General.]

**CERTIFIED COPY of an ENTRY OF DEATH**
**Pursuant to the Births and Deaths Registration Act 1953**

HC 3835

Registration District *Chester*

1953 . Death in the Sub-district of *Chester* in the *County Borough of Chester*

| No. | When and where died | Name and surname | Sex | Age | Occupation | Cause of death | Signature, description, and residence of informant | When registered | Signature of registrar |
|---|---|---|---|---|---|---|---|---|---|
| 406 | Fourteenth February 1953 City Hospital Chester us | | Male | 30 years | | 1 (a) Hyhostatic pneumonia (b) Paralysis (c) Peripheral neuritis p.m. Certified by | | Seventeenth February 1953 | RL Jarvis Registrar. |

Certified to be a true copy of an entry in a register in my custody.

K. Hanigan.

Superintendent Registrar.

14.8.95 Date.

CAUTION:—It is an offence to falsify a certificate or to make or knowingly use a false certificate or a copy of a false certificate intending it to be accepted as genuine to the prejudice of any person, or to possess a certificate knowing it to be false without lawful authority.

unaware of the family history of porphyria. His eight children are asymptomatic. Two of the four tested are positive for porphyria.

Both brothers are obligatory porphyrics, and we feel that their terminal illnesses are strongly suggestive of porphyria, possibly induced by barbiturates in the former and almost definitely by tricyclic antidepressants in the latter (Chapter 7). The fact that their death certificates (Table 3) are almost certainly incorrect has been revealed only because of our study.

Fig 3. Death certificate of subject 1.5.3.

*Deaths in the grandchildren recognised to be due to porphyria*

Five of the 16 deceased porphyric grandchildren have porphyria recorded on their death certificates.

*1.1.5*: died age 40 in 1969 in the Chester City Hospital. He was Bekerus' index case, having developed abdominal pain and red urine after an operation for nasal polyps in 1963 (see Chapter 5). His death certificate records uraemia and acute intermittent porphyria.

*1.6.5*: died age 37 in 1976 at Wrexham Maelor Hospital. He was the father of my index case, 1.6.5.3, the girl I met in the outpatient clinic in 1980 (Chapter 1) and brother of the first member (1.6.3) of the kindred to be diagnosed as having porphyria in 1954 (Chapter 4). He was called up for national service in the Royal Engineers in June 1957, but had an epileptic fit and was sent to the Royal Naval Hospital, Chatham. He was treated with phenobarbitone and developed abdominal pain, vomiting and diarrhoea. Barbiturates were stopped, and he was discharged as being medically unfit for any form of military service (letter from British Legion in Clatterbridge Hospital case-notes, Fig 3, Chapter 7). Two months later he was admitted to Clatterbridge Hospital, and acute porphyria was diagnosed after he told them the story of his sister (1.6.3) who had been treated in the same hospital for acute porphyria in 1954.

The predominant clinical features were severe abdominal pain, hallucinations and hypertension of 170/140 mmHg. His urine contained large amounts of porphobilinogen, and blood urea was raised at 102 mg% (17 mmol/l). There was muscular weakness, with tendon reflexes difficult to elicit. An EEG showed gross abnormality consistent with generalised brain damage.

He recovered, but had a porphyric crisis after a submucous resection for a nasal polyp in 1971. He was noted to have a wheezy chest in 1970. He died in 1976 about 24 hours after an emergency admission to Wrexham Maelor Hospital with severe headache. His death certificate, with the benefit of a post-mortem, recorded cerebral haemorrhage, malignant hypertension and porphyria. His eldest son (1.6.5.1), died six months later at Clatterbridge Hospital of respiratory paralysis due to porphyria and his eldest daughter (1.6.5.3), my index case, had 14 admissions with porphyric crises over the following 10 years (Chapter 7).

*1.8.3*: died age 47 in 1982 at Chester City Hospital. The house physician in her final illness records her as being a council lavatory cleaner. More prosaically, her death certificate translates her occupation as local government officer. Bekerus records that she had 'gastric sickness, backache, headache and red urine' made worse with sleeping tablets. She had a long history of hypertension, and her death certificate records renal failure and acute intermittent porphyria (see Chapter 8). She had eight children by her first marriage, four of whom are biochemically positive and one of whom (1.8.3.3) died of porphyric bulbar palsy at the age of 25. Three of her four children by the second marriage are biochemically positive.

*1.9.2*: labourer, died age 55 in 1988 in the Countess of Chester Hospital. He had abdominal pain as a younger man and later developed hypertension and chronic renal failure (see Chapter 8). He was being considered for a renal transplant when, at an unusually late age, he developed severe peripheral motor neuropathy. His death certificate records intracerebral haemorrhage, hypertension, acute intermittent porphyria and chronic renal failure. He had no children.

*1.9.3*: sister of 1.9.2, died age 22 in 1958 in Chester City Hospital. She had 'coloured urine' since the age of 14, usually premenstrually. She was sent in by her GP in the 16th week of her first pregnancy with headache and neck stiffness, with a clinical diagnosis of meningitis. She developed abdominal pain, vomiting and hypertension. Her urine was positive for porphobilinogen. The evening before she died she had an epileptic fit, and complained of difficulty swallowing thought to be due to pharyngeal paralysis. She died suddenly the next day. A post-mortem showed nothing except excess tracheal secretions. Her death certificate records acute respiratory failure and porphyria, the first certification of porphyria in the kindred (Chapter 1).

## Deaths in five known porphyric grandchildren not recorded as porphyria

Five of the remaining 21 grandchildren are known to be porphyric.

*1.1.1*: died age 63 years in 1977. Her death certificate, with the benefit of a post-mortem examination, records cerebellar haemorrhage and hypertension. She had no known porphyric symptoms, but she had obligatory porphyria and urine testing was positive in 1963.

*1.5.1*: died age 60 years in 1981. His death certificate is not available, but he died alone in a boarding house. He had a history of headaches and mental illness, and his urine was positive for porphobilinogen in the County Mental Hospital in 1963.

*1.5.2*: butcher, died age 67 years in 1988. His death certificate records ischaemic heart disease, aspiration pneumonitis and bleeding gastric ulcer. He was admitted to the Chester Royal Infirmary in 1964 with severe epigastric pain and vomiting. He was treated with propantheline and phenobarbitone; five days later he became psychotic and was transferred to the County Mental Hospital. During this admission his family history of porphyria was disclosed and his urine was strongly positive for porphobilinogen. He was given phenobarbitone as a diagnostic aid to EEG interpretation, after which he developed a further acute confusional episode which was treated with chlorpromazine. He developed some weakness of his right arm. A letter from his GP, Dr R McClure, refers to 1.5.2 labelling himself as having 'Dobson's Complaint' (Fig 8, Chapter 1) – hence the title of this book.

*1.6.3*: wife of a gas fitter, died age 46 years in 1978. Her death certificate records cerebellar haemorrhage. Post-mortem examination also showed cardiomegaly and small shrunken kidneys. She was the first person to be diagnosed as having porphyria, and her story is described in Chapter 4.

*1.6.4*: wife of a storeman, died age 58 in 1990. Her death certificate records bronchopneumonia and chronic obstructive airways disease. She was not known to have porphyric symptoms, but a blood test was positive – as is that of one of her three children.

## Deaths in four grandchildren of unknown porphyric status

*1.2.2*: died in 1982 age 62 possibly as the result of an accident but his death certificate is not available. He is the brother of the four brothers described above who died between the ages of 16 and 29.

*1.2.5*: sister of the above, died in 1986. Her death certificate is not available. She refused to cooperate with Bekerus' study.

*1.7.1*: died age 29 in 1956 in Australia. His brother tells us he died after an operation for appendicitis. Bekerus reports that porphyria was implicated, but we have no evidence for this. Two of his three children have been tested for porphyria in Australia with negative results.

*1.9.1*: wife of a steel shunter, died age 32 in 1963. Her death certificate records accidental haemorrhage (in childbirth).

### Death in one porphyria-negative grandchild

*1.1.3*: died age 72 years in 1993. After necropsy, the cause of death was given as acute cardiorespiratory failure and pneumonia.

## Generation IV: mortality in the 106 great-grandchildren

The great-grandchildren were born between 1940 and 1972. Two have died of porphyria.

*1.6.5.1*: died age 17 in 1977. He was admitted to Clatterbridge Hospital with a diagnosis of acute porphyria based on a four-day history of abdominal pain, limb pain, vomiting and red urine. The only drug prescribed by his GP was chlorpromazine. He reported that he had had milder episodes 12 and four months previously. His father (1.6.5) had died of porphyria six months before (as described earlier in the chapter), and his sister, 1.6.5.3, is our index case.

On admission, his limbs were weak and he had reduced tendon reflexes. He developed hallucinations, tachycardia and a blood pressure of 160/120 mmHg, coinciding with serum sodium falling to 121 mmol/l. Urine delta-aminolaevulinic acid was raised at 440 mmol/l (normal range 10–50 mmol/l), and urinary porphobilinogen was positive. His acute symptoms settled after treatment with chlorpromazine, propranolol and diazepam in addition to intravenous fluids (5% dextrose). After nine days he was allowed home to watch the Cup Final on television, but was readmitted with abdominal pain later the same day. It was felt that there was a degree of emotional overlay and he was given an injection of sterile water. The next day he is recorded as being weak; he managed to eat and take a bath, but was then found dead in bed. The death certificate recorded bulbar palsy and acute intermittent porphyria.

*1.8.3.3*: died age 25 in 1981. She presented in 1975 at the age of 19 years with abdominal pain, vomiting and constipation, having discontinued the oral contraceptive pill. No diagnosis was made. Her symptoms returned in 1977, at which time her mother reported the family history of porphyria. She had 16 further admissions between 1977 and her death in 1981. Her attacks all followed a common pattern of pain in the abdomen, loins and thighs, constipation, vomiting and profound misery, for which she repeatedly requested opiates. Malingering and hysteria were frequently suspected. It was noted that she had an unusual facial appearance, with marked hirsutism, acne and comedones 'almost suggestive of tuberous sclerosis', but no mention was made of photo-sensitivity. Her urine turned red on standing and contained porpho-bilinogen.

During admissions she was often noted to have raised blood pressure (up to 200/130 mmHg), blood urea (up to 30 mmol/l) and creatinine (up to 160 µmol/l), as well as hyponatraemia and hypochloraemia. On one admission she had two major seizures, which were relieved by intravenous diazepam. The fits were preceded by confusion and agitation; significantly, they occurred after an infusion over three days of 8 litre of 5% dextrose when her serum sodium was at the lowest recorded (115 mmol/l compared to 135 mmol/l on admission) (Chapter 9). At this time, her blood urea was 6.3 mmol/l, blood pressure 220/120 mmHg, and pulse 140/min.

Motor neuropathy complicated four of these admissions. In 1978, it was so severe that she could not lift her limbs against gravity. Electromyography of the biceps showed severe chronic partial degeneration with fibrillation potentials. Surprisingly, motor and sensory nerve conduction in the median, ulnar, lateral popliteal and sural nerves were normal (Chapter 7). It was two months before her muscle power returned to normal.

On her last admission she developed a progressive motor neuropathy with areflexia over a period of four days. On the fifth day she developed a bulbar palsy with dysphonia, dysarthria and profound weakness and, whilst transfer to another hospital for assisted ventilation was being considered, was found dead in bed. There was only minimal derangement of her electrolytes, with a serum sodium of 132 mmol/l, normal blood urea and creatinine levels. The death certificate records (a) bulbar palsy and (b) acute intermittent porphyria.

A menstrual history was taken on eight occasions; on five admissions the abdominal pain started about four days premenstrually. Medication was never implicated as a precipitant. There was no evidence of voluntary fasting, although her poor social circumstances and peculiar psyche might have predisposed her to this risk.

## Discussion

The striking features in this study of mortality in the family are:

- the numerous deaths in young people;
- the recurring diagnoses of hypertension, renal failure and CVA; and
- the incorrect or incomplete death certificates.

We are fortunate in having the death certificates of both Peter and Sarah Dobson, all their 10 children, 17 of 21 deceased grandchildren, and both deceased great-grandchildren. Peter and Sarah Dobson both died of cancer, but this diagnosis is not recorded as a

**Table 4.** Summary of certified causes of death in 25 porphyric subjects.

| Cause of death* | Children (7) | Grandchildren (16) | Great-grandchildren (2) | Total |
|---|---|---|---|---|
| Porphyria | 1 | 5 | 2 | 8 |
| Paralysis/bulbar palsy | 0 | 3 | 2 | 5 |
| Hypertension | 1 | 5 | 0 | 6 |
| Renal failure | 0† | 4 | 0 | 4 |
| Cerebrovascular accident | 2 | 4 | 0 | 6 |

* some subjects had more than one cause of death
† one case of uraemia and chronic urinary retention (subject 1.5) excluded

cause of death in any of their 33 deceased descendants. Kauppinen and Mustajoki reported[2,3] that death in 13 of 96 deceased porphyric subjects in Finland was due to malignancy, eight of them primary hepatocellular carcinoma (PHC). The marked occurrence of this particular cancer was first noted in Sweden.[4,5] The explanation remains obscure: patients with acute hepatic porphyrias have not been considered to be prone to any of the classical forms of liver disease, and functional and structural alterations are generally slight or absent. However, liver histology available in five of the six Swedish cases of PHC described by Andersson et al[6] all showed cirrhosis or pre-cirrhosis. The cause of the cirrhosis was not discovered – it should be noted, in particular, that alcohol consumption in porphyrics is probably less than average because it can precipitate attacks of porphyria. Batlle[7] proposed a mechanism to explain the carcinogenesis in porphyric subjects based on the reduced free haem pool. It is fortunate that the mechanism seems not to apply to Chester porphyria. Hepatoma may present as abdominal pain mimicking porphyric pain, and thus delay the diagnosis, and cytotoxic agents used to treat hepatoma may precipitate a porphyric crisis.[5]

The main causes of death of the 25 porphyric members of the kindred who have died are shown in Tables 1 and 3, and summarised in Table 4. Pneumonia is excluded, in the belief that it is often a terminal consequence of the pathological process, and to this day is often inappropriately listed as the first cause of death, contrary to advice to certifying medical practitioners.[8]

**Table 5.** Premature deaths in the kindred.

| Generation | Dates | Porphyric status | |
|---|---|---|---|
| II: 10 siblings | Born 1890–1911 Died 1938–1982 | 7 porphyric | average age at death 61 years |
| | | 3 unknown | average age at death 41 years |
| III: 38 grandchildren | Born 1913–1938 | 24 porphyric | 16 died (10 before age 50) 8 living |
| | | 9 negative | 1 died (age 72) 8 living |
| | | 5 unknown | 4 died (age 62, 58, 31, 31) 1 living |
| IV: 106 great-grandchildren | Born 1940–1972 | 25 porphyric | 2 died (age 17, 25 |
| | | 69 negative | no known deaths |
| | | 12 unknown | no known deaths |

*Life expectancy and age at death*

As previously stated, our study excludes those who died in infancy or childhood. The life expectancy of the 10 children, 38 grand-children and 106 great-grandchildren is summarised in Table 5. The relatively young age of death in several subjects may partially explain the absence of cancer deaths.

*Generation II.* The life expectancy of the 10 siblings (average age at death 55 years) is probably little less than that expected for people born around the turn of the century. At first sight, the causes of death (Table 1) in the 10 siblings give little evidence that por-phyria runs in the family and is destined to blight the life expectancy of the next generation. Only subject 1.9 was certified as dying from porphyria, and she had a history of agitation and abdominal and back pain. Without the medical records it is impossible to know whether porphyria was responsible for some of the premature deaths in the siblings who died before the antibiotic era: 1.1, 1.7 and 1.8 died of pneumonia at the ages of 48, 36 and 32 years. It is frus-trating that the case-notes of subject 1.7 from the County Mental Hospital, which we do have, do not record whether barbiturates were used to treat the confusional insanity or pains in the head. His history is similar to that of his nephew, 1.2.8, who died age 18 years shortly after leaving the same hospital, and also reminiscent of the psychoses precipitated by barbiturates in some other grandchildren, particularly subjects 1.5.2 and 1.6.3 (Chapter 4). The youngest sibling, 1.10, died aged 38 years of coronary thrombosis in 1949, but Bekerus was told he had paralysis of his arms.

It is difficult to resist the speculation that the three siblings of unknown status were in fact porphyric. The brothers 1.7 and 1.10, as mentioned above, both died in their 30s, and their sister, 1.3, died age 49 of uraemia and hypertension – both conditions strongly linked to porphyria in our kindred (Chapter 8). Neither 1.3 nor 1.10 had children who reached adulthood, so the speculation remains unanswered. Two of the three children of 1.7 tested were negative for porphyria.

*Generation III.* It is evident from Table 3 that porphyria blighted the life expectancy of the 38 grandchildren. One family lost four sons, aged 16, 18, 21 and 29 years, between 1941 and 1953. These four had no issue, and they are the only subjects in our study in whom the label of porphyria is given on circumstantial evidence. A surviving brother (1.2.6) has positive blood tests, so their father (1.2) is an obligatory carrier.

Hypertension and CVA were each implicated in six deaths of the grandchildren, and renal failure in four. In an ordinary population with a normal life expectancy this might not be remarkable, but eight grandchildren died of these conditions at the ages of 63, 40, 29, 18, 46, 37, 47 and 55 years (in notation order) (Table 3). Significantly, all four grandchildren suffering a CVA had necropsies: in two (1.1.1, 1.6.3) cerebellar haemorrhage was shown, and in two (1.6.5, 1.9.2) cerebral haemorrhage, suggesting that these events were related to hypertension, as opposed to the thrombotic strokes commoner in the elderly. Necropsy reports are available for subjects 1.6.3 and 1.9.2, and both showed small shrunken kidneys (Chapter 8). Many of the living grandchildren have hypertension, which we can be sure is a marker for porphyria as porphyria-negative grandchildren are not affected (Chapter 8). If this is true, it lends weight to the speculation that subject 1.3, of unknown porphyria status, whose death certificate records uraemia and hypertension (Table 1), might have been porphyric.

The prevalence of hypertension and renal failure in other series is discussed in Chapter 8. Surprisingly, CVA is not mentioned as a cause of death in 96 porphyric subjects described by Kauppinen and Mustajoki,[3] in view of the fact that 18% of their 158 living subjects had hypertension. Similarly, the prevalence of strokes in 50 porphyric subjects described by Andersson and Lithner[9] was no different from matched controls, despite a 27% prevalence of hypertension in the porphyric subjects.

*Incorrect or incomplete death certificates*

Our knowledge of the medical histories of the 10 siblings is scanty. In trying to decide whether a subject could have been porphyric, it is difficult to balance the need for scientific rigour against the temptation to speculate. Rimington (quoted in Ref 10) warned that, when attributing porphyria to a deceased person, the most that should be done is to formulate a hypothesis which *may* be corroborated by evidence but may never be proved. (He was co-author of the paper in the *British Medical Journal* in 1968[11] which claimed that King George III had variegate porphyria, an assertion which was scorned by many porphyria experts across the world.)

Seven of the 10 siblings are obligatory porphyrics as their children are affected. As mentioned above, subject 1.3 died of uraemia and hypertension, and in the next generation these conditions are certainly linked to the porphyric grandchildren but not to their porphyria-negative cousins. Thus, the death certificate of 1.3 may be incomplete. We have speculated similarly with subjects 1.7 and 1.10.

We have described the sad deaths of the four young brothers, 1.2.1, 1.2.3, 1.2.4 and 1.2.8, the only cases in our kindred in which speculation has triumphed over caution and the porphyric designation rests on circumstantial evidence. If we are right in our assumptions, incorrect or incomplete death certificates have been issued for these subjects. Bekerus was told that the first three brothers were paralysed. We feel sure the death certificates of all four brothers are incomplete with respect to porphyria. Their deaths were registered as follows:

*1.2.1*: certified as dying from uraemia, nephritis and mental deficiency – conditions common in several other cousins.

*1.2.3*: the intriguing diagnosis of myotonia atrophica as the cause of death – obviously a reflection of the paralysis (Fig 2).

*1.2.4*: the third brother in whom the family remember paralysis, died of pneumonia after an operation for 'appendicitis' age 16. We suspect that he may have been operated on for porphyric pain, and that his paralysis may have been precipitated either by the barbiturate anaesthetic induction agent or by subsequently prescribed barbiturates, as in the cases of his cousins, 1.5.2 and 1.9.5 (Chapter 7).

*1.2.8*: the fourth brother, not remembered to have been paralysed, died of left ventricular failure and malignant hypertension 12 days after discharge from the County Mental Hospital.

The death certificates of two brothers in a different family tell the same story:

*1.5.3*: an obligatory carrier, is certified as dying from hypostatic pneumonia, paralysis and peripheral neuritis (Fig 3).

*1.5.5*: his brother, and also an obligatory carrier, presented with psychosis, apparent meningitis and then coma, yet nothing definitive was found at necropsy. The pathologist's ingenuity must have been taxed to attribute death to acute heart failure, atherosclerosis and bronchitis. We are sure the death was porphyric. Two cases of sudden 'cerebral' death in acute intermittent porphyria are recorded by Stein and Tschudy.[12]

The pathologist concerned with the necropsy of subject 1.6.3 was more economical with the facts. Although the history of porphyria-related malignant hypertension, uraemia, paralysis and psychosis was known from 1954, the death certificate only records cerebellar haemorrhage and omits porphyria – a further example of an incomplete death certificate (Fig 2, Chapter 4).

Thus, seven of the 16 porphyric grandchildren who have died, all of them under the age of 52, have incomplete or incorrect death certificates. It is hardly surprising that this premature mortality resulted in anguish and fear in the kindred, and that during our enquiries over the years some have denied that the 'taint' affects their branch of the family. Three siblings of the four brothers who died in their teens and 20s refused to cooperate with Bekerus. Family confidence was further marred when symptomatic members were suspected of hysteria (1.6.3, 1.1.1.1, 1.6.5.1, Chapter 11) or when, despite warnings of the family history by her husband, subject 1.9.5 was given a barbiturate anaesthetic and developed a porphyric crisis resulting in coma (Chapter 7). We hope that family confidence is slowly being restored as it is eight years since the last porphyria-related death (1.9.2), but some family members are understandably frustrated by equivocal biochemical tests of their porphyria status. We look forward to genetic tests of the diagnosis.

*Mortality in other series*

Eales[13] quotes a 22% death rate in the acute attack, Mustajoki and Koskelo[14] 30%, and Goldberg[15] a 25% death rate within five years of the acute attack. Death rates are highest in the second and third decade and if there has been neurological involvement. Beattie and Goldberg[16] reported a 57% survival 20 years after onset of the acute attack, and attributed the declining mortality rate of recent years to improvements in intensive care therapy and withdrawal of previous precipitating factors. Kauppinen and Mustajoki[3] recorded that 31 of 96 of their deceased porphyric subjects had died of porphyria itself, but none since 1979.

*Post-mortem examinations*

Reports of necropsy in cases of acute intermittent porphyria[17,18] and variegate porphyria[19] are not common. The findings in all three reported studies were diverse, non-specific, and included peripheral nerve pathology which is now thought to represent mainly axonal degeneration[20,21] (see also Chapter 7). We have necropsy reports on only five members in our series:

*1.5.5*: died after a history of psychosis, meningism and coma, with no explanation found at necropsy.

*1.1.1, 1.6.3, 1.6.5, 1.9.2*: died with intracranial haemorrhage, the second and fourth with small shrunken kidneys (following a history of hypertension and renal failure).

We have no histological reports on nerve tissue from subjects dying of paralysis.

## References

1 Qadiri MR, Church SE, McColl KEL, Moore MR, Youngs GR. Chester porphyria: a clinical study of a new form of acute porphyria. *British Medical Journal* 1986; **292**: 455–9.

2 Kauppinen R, Mustajoki P. Acute hepatic porphyria and hepatocellular carcinoma. *British Journal of Cancer* 1988; **57**: 117–20.

3 Kauppinen R, Mustajoki P. Prognosis of acute porphyria: occurrence of acute attacks, precipitating factors and associated diseases. *Medicine* 1992; **71**: 1–13.

4 Hardell L, Bengtsson NO, Jonsson U, Eriksson S, Larsson LG. Aetiological aspects on primary liver cell cancer with special regard to alcohol, organic solvents and acute intermittent porphyria – an epidemiological investigation. *British Journal of Cancer* 1984; **50**: 389–97.

5 Lithner F, Wetterberg L. Hepatocellular carcinoma in patients with acute intermittent porphyria. *Acta Medica Scandinavica* 1984; **215**: 271–4.

6 Andersson C, Bjersing L, Lithner F. The epidemiology of hepatocellular carcinoma in patients with acute intermittent porphyria. *Journal of Internal Medicine* 1996; **240**: 195–201.

7 Batlle AM. Porphyrins, porphyrias, cancer and photodynamic therapy – a model for carcinogenesis. *Journal of Photochemistry and Photobiology* 1993; **20**: 5–22.

8 *Medical certificates of cause of death*. London: Her Majesty's Stationery Office, 1995.

9 Andersson C, Lithner F. Hypertension and renal disease in patients with acute intermittent porphyria. *Journal of Internal Medicine* 1994; **236**: 169–75.

10 Dean G. *The porphyrias, a story of inheritance and environment*, 2nd edn. London: Pitman, 1971.

11 Macalpine I, Hunter R, Rimington C. Porphyria in the Royal Houses of Stuart, Hanover, and Prussia. A follow-up study of George III's illness. *British Medical Journal* 1968; **1**: 7–18.

12  Stein JA, Tschudy JP. Acute intermittent porphyria. A clinical and bio-chemical study of 46 patients. *Medicine* 1970; **49**: 1–16.

13  Eales L. Porphyria as seen in Cape Town. A survey of 250 cases and some recent studies. *South African Journal of Laboratory and Clinical Medicine* 1963; **9**: 151–62.

14  Mustajoki P, Koskelo P. Hereditary hepatic porphyrias in Finland. *Acta Medica Scandinavica* 1976; **200**: 171–8.

15  Goldberg A. Acute intermittent porphyria: a study of 50 cases. *Quarterly Journal of Medicine* 1959; **28**: 183–209.

16  Beattie AD, Goldberg A. Acute intermittent porphyria. Natural history and prognosis. In: Doss M (ed). *Porphyrias and human diseases*. Basel: Karger, 1976.

17  Gibson JB, Goldberg A. The neuropathology of acute porphyria. *Journal of Pathology and Bacteriology* 1956; **71**: 495–509.

18  Ten Eyck FW, Martin WJ, Kernohan JW. Acute porphyria: necropsy studies in nine cases. *Proceedings of the Staff Meetings of the Mayo Clinic* 1961; **36**: 409–22.

19  Campbell JAH. The pathology of the South African genetic porphyria. *South African Journal of Laboratory and Clinical Medicine* 1963; **9**: 197–203.

20  Bonkowsky HL, Schady W. Neurologic manifestations of acute porphyria. *Seminars in Liver Disease* 1982; **2**: 108–24.

21  Yamada M, Kondo M, Tanaka M, Okeda R, *et al*. An autopsy case of acute porphyria with a decrease of both uroporphyrinogen-1-synthetase and ferrochelatase activities. *Acta Neuropathologica* 1984; **64**: 6–11.

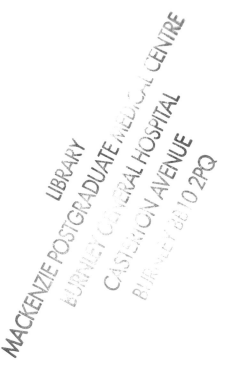

*Chapter 7*

# Morbidity in the kindred: a story of missed or delayed diagnoses

GILES YOUNGS AND MOHAMMAD QADIRI

Waldenström recognised the variability of the clinical manifestations of acute porphyria in 1939,[1] and likened it to syphilis as deserving the epithet *la petite simulatrice*. Included in his long list of differential diagnoses for the neurological manifestations of acute porphyria were: encephalitis, poliomyelitis, myelitis, radial nerve palsy, polyneuritis, polyarteritis nodosa, cerebral tumour, progressive muscular atrophy, lead or arsenic poisoning, psychoneurosis and hysteria. The widespread pains, curious pareses and emotional disturbances with only vague physical signs and normal investigations have often been mistaken for hysteria. In 1963, Gajdos and Gajdos-Török[2] reported a 46% frequency of diagnostic error of the acute porphyric attack. Goldberg and Rimington[3] had suggested in the previous year that the entire spectrum of symptoms of the acute episode (including abdominal, neurological, psychiatric and autonomic) is explicable on a neurogenic basis. The clinical manifestations of porphyria in the Chester kindred, especially in the 38 grandchildren, have also presented as a cornucopia of syndromes to general practitioners (GPs) and hospital clinicians of many specialties (Table 1), with the unsurprising consequence of delayed diagnosis and incorrect death certificates.

## Manifestation of porphyria in relation to age and gender

The 17 members of generation III (grandchildren) who experienced abdominal pain were symptomatic mainly between their late teens and early 30s, which is in keeping with other published series. We do not know of any prepubertal members of the family who have had symptomatic porphyria. Subject 1.2.4 died in 1941 after an operation for 'appendicitis' at the age of 16. He is remembered

Table 1. Twenty-four porphyric grandchildren: spectrum of hospital presentations with symptoms or complications of porphyria.

| Subject | Sex | Symptomatic (S) or latent (L) | Age at presentation (years) | Morbidity and mortality |
|---------|-----|-------------------------------|-----------------------------|-------------------------|
| *General physicians* | | | | |
| 1.1.1 | F | L | 63 | Cerebellar haemorrhage. Hypertension |
| 1.1.6 | F | L | 35 | Hypertension. Chronic renal failure |
| 1.2.1 | M | S | 29 | Uraemia. Nephritis |
| 1.2.3 | M | S | 21 | Myotonia atrophica |
| 1.4.1 | M | L | 59 | Hypertension |
| 1.5.3 | M | S | 30 | Paralysis. Peripheral neuritis |
| 1.5.5 | M | S | 51 | Meningism and coma after tricyclic antidepressant |
| 1.6.1 | M | S | 40 | Abdominal pain. Hypertension |
| 1.6.3 | F | S | 23 | Malignant hypertension. Paralysis. Psychosis |
| 1.6.5 | M | S | 20 | Porphyric crisis. Epileptic seizure |
| 1.8.1 | M | S | ? | Hypertension. Renal failure |
| 1.8.2 | M | S | 37 | Hypertension. Renal failure. Abdominal pain |
| 1.9.2 | M | S | 44 | Hypertension. Renal failure. Peripheral neuropathy |
| 1.9.3 | F | S | 22 | Meningism. Bulbar palsy |
| *General surgeons* | | | | |
| 1.2.4 | M | S | 16 | Post-operative death. Paralysed legs |
| 1.5.2 | M | S | 43 | Abdominal pain, then psychosis |
| 1.6.1 | M | S | 18 | Abdominal pain |
| 1.8.1 | M | S | ? | Abdominal pain |
| *Obstetricians/gynaecologists* | | | | |
| 1.6.3 | F | S | 29 | Porphyric crisis in pregnancy |
| 1.8.3 | F | S | 31 | Pregnancy and post-partum hypertension |
| 1.9.5 | F | S | 27 | Post-operative porphyric crisis. Psychosis |
| *Psychiatrists: admission to County Mental Hospital* | | | | |
| 1.2.8 | M | S | 18 | Psychosis. Died 12 days after discharge |
| 1.5.1 | M | S | 42 | Depression. Suicidal |
| 1.5.2 | M | S | 43 | Post-operative psychosis |
| 1.5.5 | M | S | 50 | Depression and self neglect |
| 1.6.3 | F | S | 23 | Post-barbiturate psychosis |
| 1.8.2 | M | S | 40 | Paranoid delusions |
| *Ear, nose and throat surgeons* | | | | |
| 1.1.5 | M | S | 35 | Post-operative porphyric crisis |
| 1.6.5 | M | S | 33 | Post-operative porphyric crisis |

Seven subjects appear under more than one heading because either they presented to different departments on separate occasions or the complication of their porphyric crisis necessitated transfer to another department. There are no neurological beds in Chester, and only one subject (1.6.3) was transferred to neurological care. Of the six grandchildren with latent porphyria, three have hypertension (1.1.1, 1.1.6, 1.4.1), and are therefore listed above; the other three (1.2.6, 1.6.2, 1.6.4) are not listed because they have not presented to hospital with symptoms or complications of porphyria.

to have had paralysed legs (Chapter 6), and we suspect he may have undergone laparotomy for porphyric pain, which was followed by paralysis because of barbiturate administration. Three great-grandchildren (1.6.5.1, 1.6.5.3, 1.8.3.3) presented at the age of 16, 15 and 19 years, respectively. Subjects 1.8.1 and 1.9.2 (Chapter 8) had their last acute attacks at the age of 44 and 54 years, respectively. The porphyria-related morbidity and mortality of the older age groups are due to complications of hypertension and renal failure (Chapters 6 and 8).

An individual with latent porphyria is one who has never manifested symptoms of porphyria but has positive biochemical tests or obligatory porphyria because his or her children are porphyric. Latency is not easy to define because abdominal pain (eg irritable bowel syndrome[4]) is common in the general population, while there is no reliable laboratory marker to prove an episode of mild pain is due to porphyria.

Assays for the deficient enzyme (porphobilinogen deaminase in acute intermittent porphyria) are often inconclusive, with large overlap zones between normal and porphyric subjects.[5,6] Urinary porphobilinogen is often absent in latent porphyria, so is of limited value as a screening test.

We believe that six of the 24 (25%) porphyric grandchildren (1.1.1, 1.1.6, 1.2.6, 1.4.1, 1.6.2, 1.6.4) and 15 of the 25 (60%) great-grandchildren (generation IV) have latent porphyria (43% latency for the two generations combined) (Table 2). The greater risk of symptomatic porphyria in the senior generation is largely due to inappropriate medications. Two recent studies in Finland[7] and Sweden[8] show the prevalence of latency to be 66% and 50% respectively, rather less than in Scotland where:

> the vast majority of patients with the genetic trait for acute intermittent porphyria are clinically latent.[6]

Table 2 also shows that in our kindred symptomatic porphyria is significantly more common in males than in females ($\chi^2 = 6.84$; $p < 0.01$). Church et al[9,10] showed that latency does not protect against the hypertension and chronic renal failure believed to be complications of porphyria.

*1.1.1*: certified to have died of cerebellar haemorrhage and hypertension.

*1.1.6*: his sister, currently has advanced chronic renal failure and hypertension (Chapter 8). Neither had symptoms of acute porphyria.

Church et al[9,10] also found mean blood pressure to be higher in 17 latent porphyric subjects than in 23 non-porphyric members of the family (Chapter 8).

**Table 2.** Symptomatic and latent porphyria in relation to gender.

| | No. at risk | Porphyria | | | Not tested |
| | | Symptomatic | Latent | Porphyria-negative | |
|---|---|---|---|---|---|
| **Generation III** | | 35 (92%) of 38 grandchildren have a porphyric parent | | | |
| | | 24 (77%) of the 31 tested inherited porphyria | | | |
| Male | 19 | 14 | 2 | 2 | 1 |
| Female | 16 | 4 | 4 | 5 | 3 |
| *Subtotal* | *35* | *18* | *6* | *7* | *4* |
| **Generation IV** | | 58 (55%) of 106 great-grandchildren have a porphyric parent | | | |
| | | 25 (52%) of the 48 tested inherited porphyria | | | |
| Male | 32 | 6 | 5 | 14 | 7 |
| Female | 26 | 4 | 10 | 9 | 3 |
| *Subtotal* | *58* | *10* | *15* | *23* | *10* |
| **Both generations** | | 93 (65%) of 144 offspring have a porphyric parent | | | |
| | | 49 (62%) of the 79 tested inherited porphyria | | | |
| Male | 51 | 20* | 7* | 16 | 8 |
| Female | 42 | 8* | 14* | 14 | 6 |
| *Total* | *93* | *28* | *21* | *30* | *14* |

*$\chi^2 = 6.84$; $p < 0.01$

Symptomatic porphyria is significantly more common in male than in female members of the Chester family.

## The acute attack

Clinical details of generation II (10 siblings) are scanty. Subject 1.3 died age 48 years in 1942. She lodged with her sister (1.4) for a while during the war, whose son (1.4.1) told us that his aunt died suddenly after suffering abdominal pain. Her brother (1.5) was investigated for abdominal pain in 1963 and 1967, with negative results. Bekerus was told he had headaches, bowel problems, abdominal and back pain, and that he was stubborn and bad tempered. He was one of the last of the family to live by the River Dee. His GP, Dr Vincent Tonge, wrote in 1977:

> He lives in a rather rickety house down by the Dee where he is looked after by an old female companion. He is wearing two heavy rows of war medals – perhaps Jubilee week* has reactivated old grievances about lack of a war pension.

The psychiatric notes of another brother (1.7) record 'severe pains in the head' – a common symptom in porphyric subjects. The

*The twenty-fifth jubilee of the accession to the throne of Her Majesty Queen Elizabeth II.

sisters (1.8, 1.9) were both said to have a history of abdominal and back pain.

Eighteen of the 24 porphyric grandchildren (75%) and eight of the 25 porphyric great-grandchildren (32%) have had acute illnesses which we believe were due to porphyria. One great-grandchild (1.8.3.3) had 17 admissions between 1975 and 1981, when she died age 25 while awaiting transfer for ventilation for bulbar palsy (Chapter 6). Her second cousin, 1.6.5.3, the teenage girl I met in outpatients in 1980 (Chapter 1) had 14 admissions between 1981 and 1985. The attacks in both subjects (31 admissions in all) followed a common pattern. On arrival in hospital, the predominant feature was pain in the abdomen, loins and thighs. In addition, there was often constipation, vomiting, profound distress and misery, with frequent pleas for opiate injections. Malingering and hysteria were frequently suspected by both nursing and medical staff. A menstrual history was taken on 15 of the 31 admissions; this revealed that the attack preceded menstruation by about four days. Medication was never implicated. The features of the 31 episodes are compared with the findings of previous workers in Table 3.

The management of the acute attack is difficult and unsatisfactory. The patients' frequent pleas for opiates cause conflict with both medical and nursing staff. The misery and anxiety are unrelated to any electrolyte disturbance. Oral analgesia is often not tolerated, and intramuscular injections may cause painful induration of the buttocks. Latterly, we have used syringe drivers by the subcutaneous or intravenous route. In a particularly severe attack, subject 1.6.5.3 was admitted for 40 days and needed a total of 9,320 mg of opiates (7,850 mg in 131 separate injections of pethidine, plus 1,470 mg as morphine suppositories). Subjects 1.6.5.3 and 1.8.3.3

Table 3. Percentage incidence of clinical features of acute porphyric crisis.

| | Waldenström[11] (1957) | Goldberg[12] (1959) | Markovitz[13] (1954) | Eales[14] (1962) | Church[9] (1986) |
|---|---|---|---|---|---|
| No. of cases | 233 | 50 | 69 | 80 | 31* |
| *Percentage incidence* | | | | | |
| Abdominal pain | 85 | 94 | 95 | 90 | 100 |
| Epilepsy | 10 | 18 | — | 12 | 6 |
| Paralysis | 42 | 68 | 72 | 53 | 30 |
| Psychological disturbance | 55 | 56 | 80 | 55 | 100 |
| Tachycardia | 28 | 64 | 51 | 83 | 78 |
| Hypertension | 40 | 56 | 49 | 55 | 30 |

*31 admissions in two subjects.

both had an epileptic fit; this was associated with a serum sodium of 115 mmol/l, and probably related to overinfusion of 5% dextrose solution (Chapter 9).

The advice to administer a high carbohydrate intake[15] is difficult to follow because of the invariable nausea, the propensity of concentrated dextrose solutions to damage veins, and the danger of 5% dextrose leading to severe hyponatraemia. We have little experience of haematin or hormone manipulation as their inception coincided with a sudden reduction in admissions of our family members with acute crises. In hospital, motor neuropathy is monitored four times a day with tests of finger abduction and peak expiratory flow rate. Subject 1.6.5.3 developed a severe motor neuropathy on two occasions which took some months to recover. She had only occasional mild crises needing hospital admission between 1985 and 1990, and has remained well since. More details of the story of her second cousin (1.8.3.3) are given in Chapter 6.

## Precipitating factors

### Surgery

Three subjects (1.1.5, 1.6.5, 1.9.5) developed porphyric crises after surgical procedures and a fourth (1.2.4), described above, died after post-operative paralysis. The first two underwent surgery for nasal polyps. Thiopentone, a barbiturate used for inducing anaesthesia for 60 years, was used in subject 1.1.5 (Chapter 5) and probably in the other two cases. The third subject (1.9.5) had no history of porphyric symptoms, but warned her medical advisers of the family history of porphyria before she underwent surgical sterilisation. She developed a porphyric crisis with psychiatric disturbance post-operatively, and her husband refused transfer to the County Mental Hospital. She became comatose for three days, and subsequent tests for porphyria were positive. Subject 1.7.1, of unknown porphyria status, died after an appendicectomy in Australia age 29 years, but no further details are known.

Surgery has long been recognised as a hazard in people with acute hepatic porphyria and, as abdominal pain is the commonest symptom of the acute porphyrias, subjects are at risk of having exploratory laparotomies. This was particularly true in previous decades before modern radiological diagnostic aids became available. Other perioperative risks include metabolic stress, especially hyponatraemia, starvation and infection. Several authors[11,16,17] describe porphyric crises, sometimes ending in death, after surgery – in some cases performed inappropriately for porphyric abdominal pain. The main hazard is in subjects hitherto unknown to have porphyria. Dover *et al*[17] described 29 operations in 19 patients known to have porphyria, with no deaths or porphyric crises. Propofol was the most commonly used intravenous anaesthetic agent, confirming a previous prospective study of its safety in variegate porphyria.[18] This echoes our experience in Chester where, since the experience of subject 1.9.5 15 years ago, there has been no post-operative porphyric crisis in a family member. In a retrospective study of 158 subjects with acute porphyria in Finland, Kauppinen and Mustajoki[7] found only three of 163 surgical operations were followed by porphyric attacks. Dover *et al*[17] highlight that a further hazard people with porphyria may meet is of being denied surgery lest a porphyric crisis ensue! They quote the case of a woman denied breast lumpectomy who later presented with extensive local and metastatic malignancy making surgery mandatory. This outcome might have been avoided by earlier and less mutilating surgery.

*Barbiturates and other drugs*

Porphyric pain may be confused with irritable bowel syndrome,[19] for which Chaudhary and Truelove in their landmark paper on this condition in 1962[20] recommended phenobarbitone, 65 mg once or twice daily. In a double-blind trial in patients with irritable bowel syndrome, Kasich and Rafsky in 1959[21] had found that the combination of phenobarbitone with an anticholinergic drug was better than either drug alone.

Barbiturates were widely used in psychiatric practice. Details of eight subjects who received barbiturates in association with psychiatric illness are listed in Table 1, Chapter 11. They may have contributed to the death of subject 1.7 (porphyria status unknown) who died in the County Mental Hospital age 36 years (Chapter 6). The first member of the kindred (1.6.3) to be diagnosed as having acute porphyria presented in 1954 with malignant hypertension. She developed acute psychosis and paralysis after barbiturate treatment (Chapter 4). Her cousin, 1.5.2, developed an acute abdomen in 1962 for which he was given phenobarbitone. He developed a confusional state which became worse when the drug was again administered as an aid to EEG diagnosis. We believe the psychosis and subsequent meningism, coma and death of his brother, 1.5.5, followed by normal necropsy appearances, was a porphyria-related death precipitated by tricyclic antidepressants which are known to be unsafe in acute porphyria[15,22] (Chapter 11). The fact that he was an obligatory carrier of porphyria was established only during our study. Subject 1.9.2 developed a severe peripheral neuropathy shortly after starting aluminium hydroxide, a drug listed as being unsafe in porphyria[15,22] for his advanced renal failure (Chapter 8).

*Alcohol and smoking*

Acute ingestion of alcohol can trigger porphyric crises, but only one of our subjects (1.8.1) gave a clear history of this, and there is no other evidence of alcoholism in the family. Cigarette smoking has also been implicated as a trigger.[23] As part of our atopy study (Chapter 10) a smoking history was taken from the 45 adult members who took part: 13 of 21 (62%) with porphyria were smokers, and 12 of 24 (50%) without porphyria. There was no difference between those with symptomatic and latent porphyria.

## Hypertension and renal failure

Hypertension (defined as diastolic blood pressure >100 mmHg) is common and often labile in the acute attack of porphyria. Table 3 shows a prevalence of about 50% in over 400 patients; in the 31 admissions in our two young women, the rate was 30%. More importantly, many of the premature deaths in our kindred were found to be due to chronic hypertension and renal failure[9,10] – a little reported, long-standing complication of porphyria. Many living members with porphyria, but not their porphyria-negative siblings, are also afflicted: 62% of the 16 porphyric grandchildren tested had hypertension and 50% of 14 porphyric grandchildren had renal impairment, all of whom were also hypertensive (Chapter 8). It is by no means certain that the renal failure is secondary to hypertension, as illustrated by our index case (1.6.5.3) who had 14 hospital admissions with transitory hypertension and uraemia, but who in 1995 and 1997 was normotensive (130/85 mmHg), with mildly raised blood urea (8.7 and 7.5 mmol/l) and creatinine (132 and 126 µmol/l). (Other similar cases are quoted in Chapter 8.)

## Neurological complications

In generation II, two brothers (1.1, 1.10) are remembered to have had paralysis, although this is not mentioned on their death certificates (Chapter 6). Eleven of the 24 porphyric siblings are known to have had paralysis:

*1.2.1*: died age 29 in 1946 of uraemia, acute nephritis and mental deficiency. There is a strong family memory that he was paralysed.

*1.2.3*: his brother, died age 21 years in 1943 of 'myotonia atrophica'. Bekerus was told he had paralysed legs.

*1.2.4*: another brother, died age 16 years in 1941 of pneumonia and operation (appendicitis). Bekerus was told he had paralysed legs.

Porphyria was not recorded on the death certificates of any of these three (Chapter 6).

*1.5.2*: developed weakness in the right arm after phenobarbitone treatment for abdominal pain, and subsequently as an aid to EEG interpretation (Chapter 6).

*1.5.3*: his brother, died age 30 years in 1953 of pneumonia, paralysis and peripheral neuritis (Fig 3, Chapter 6). His obligatory porphyria carrier status was discovered only as a result of this study.

*1.5.5*: another brother, died after developing muscular weakness, bulbar palsy, meningism and finally coma. His case is described more fully in Chapter 6. His obligatory carrier status was also discovered only in this study.

*1.6.1*: developed muscular weakness during one of his porphyric crises.

*1.6.3*: his sister, developed flaccid paralysis after barbiturate treatment for malignant hypertension (Chapter 4).

*1.6.5*: their brother, was admitted to Clatterbridge Hospital with acute porphyric crisis in 1958 at the age of 20 years; he developed weakness, especially abduction of shoulders, extension of the wrists and hip flexion (Chapter 6).

*1.9.2*: developed a severe peripheral motor neuropathy at the unusually late age of 54 years, which detained him in hospital for six months (Chapter 8).

*1.9.3*: his sister, died age 22 in 1958 after a short illness of neck stiffness, abdominal pain and pharyngeal paralysis (Chapter 6).

Peripheral neuropathy has had serious consequences in the few members of generation IV who have suffered porphyric crises:

*1.6.5.1* and *1.8.3.3*: both died of bulbar palsy age 17 and 25, respectively (Chapter 6).

*1.6.5.3*: 14 admissions with acute crises, and developed a severe motor neuropathy on two occasions which took several months to clear.

In summary, 14 porphyric members of the kindred have developed neuropathy, at least six of these proceeding to bulbar palsy which caused death in at least four (1.5.3, 1.9.3, 1.6.5.1, 1.8.3.3). Bulbar palsy may also have caused the death of subject 1.2.3 ('myotonia atrophica') (Fig 2, Chapter 6) and possibly his two brothers (1.2.1, 1.2.4), both of whom are remembered to have been paralysed in their terminal illnesses in the 1940s, although this is not mentioned on the death certificates.

The neuropathy in all the cases we have observed is predominantly motor, with consequent weakness and muscle wasting. The major sensory component is pain rather than paraesthesia or loss of sensation, which is in keeping with the experience of others.[1,24,25]

It is difficult to explain the normal motor and sensory nerve conduction in subject 1.8.3.3 when she was paralysed (Chapter 6). A similar phenomenon was reported by Ridley in his case 21.[24] In a literature review, Bonkowsky and Schady[25] found only 25% of patients with flaccid paralysis had slowing of motor conduction. These authors also review the conflicting evidence for demyelination or axonal degeneration being the pathogenetic lesion, and speculate about possible toxic agents, delta-aminolaevulinic acid being the chief suspect. Overproduction of this substance may mimic the effects of gamma-aminobutyric acid and cause the reduction in plasma melatonin levels observed in acute porphyria.[26] Many authors[1,12,14,24] have found a large proportion of neuropathic cases to be associated with barbiturate medication, but it must be remembered that medication was not implicated in the severe attacks of neuropathy in subjects 1.6.5.3 and 1.8.3.3.

The pathogenesis of neurological dysfunction in the acute porphyria syndromes remains elusive, but more may be learnt following the description of the first animal model of acute hepatic porphyria by Meyer's group.[27] Their genetically engineered mouse has porphobilinogen deaminase deficiency which recapitulates both the drug-induced biochemical abnormalities of acute hepatic porphyria and the neurological manifestations.

## Intracerebral pathology

The six deaths due to cerebrovascular accidents, shown to be haemorrhage in the four necropsies performed, are discussed in Chapter 6, as is that of 1.5.5 who died after developing papilloedema, meningism and coma, but whose necropsy failed to explain the cause. He was normotensive and normonatraemic throughout, demonstrating that the mechanisms of porphyric encephalopathy are uncertain. Wetterberg[28] named the phenomenon 'organic brain syndrome' (the subject has recently been reviewed by Sze[29]).

## Retinal abnormalities

Papilloedema has been documented in four subjects:

> *1.2.8*: died age 18 in 1953 shortly after discharge from the County Mental Hospital. His death certificate recorded malignant hypertension.

> *1.5.5*: his cousin, died with papilloedema, meningism and coma, but was normotensive (Chapter 6).

*1.6.3*: had malignant hypertension and suffered transient blindness (her story is told in Chapter 4).

*1.6.5*: her brother, died after a very short illness of headache. His death certificate records cerebral haemorrhage, malignant hypertension and porphyria (Chapter 6).

Retinal abnormalities were seen in two other porphyric subjects. Subject 1.6.5.2 (son of 1.6.5), is biochemically positive for porphyria; he is normotensive, has recurrent headaches, but only occasional abdominal and loin pain. Because of his father's terminal symptoms, I examined his optic fundi in 1985, when he was aged 23 years. They were abnormal, so I referred him to Mr S Armstrong, consultant ophthalmologist, who found that he had bilateral swollen optic discs, which were pale with no haemorrhages and reminiscent of optic nerve drusen. Computed tomography brain scan was normal, and there was no change in the ophthalmoscopic appearances three and nine months later. He remains well apart from intermittent headaches.

Subject 1.9.2 presented with failing vision in 1977, and was found to have scattered retinal haemorrhages in both eyes. There were no exudates or papilloedema. Mr JF Cogan, consultant ophthalmologist, wrote:

> these (haemorrhages) do occur in this condition (porphyria) and this must be the cause as his blood pressure is normal and there is no evidence of diabetes.

At this time, he had mild renal failure and hyperuricaemia (Chapter 8, Part 3), and a normal glucose tolerance test. His blood pressure was 140/80 mmHg on two occasions but became raised two years later, by which time his renal function was more seriously compromised. His retinal haemorrhages persisted, and in the two years before his death in 1988 he had several vitreous haemorrhages.

Ocular complications of acute hepatic porphyria are scantily reported in the literature. They are not mentioned in the 1987 monograph by Moore et al,[15] although this group had published a retinal photograph of exudative hypertensive retinopathy.[30] In his series of 50 cases Goldberg[12] described one patient with papilloedema, hypertension and fits, and four with retinal artery spasm. Amblyopia has been ascribed to angiospastic phenomena, usually in the hypertensive phase of a porphyric crisis, by many authors.[31,32] The nine cases described by Waldenström[11] experienced transitory amblyopia, while a case reported by DeFrancisco et al[33] developed optic atrophy, probably due to infarction of the optic nerve. Barnes and Boshoff[34] noted two types of retinal oedema during acute 'cerebral episodes' of variegate porphyria. The optic disc on occasion was 'hazy and slightly swollen'. Haemorrhages were seen in only one patient, and there is no mention of blood pressure or of frank papilloedema. More recently, Meier's group[35] has described two patients with cortical blindness accompanied by extensive lesions of the occipital white matter on magnetic resonance imaging, consistent with vasospasm-induced ischaemia. Neither subject had the classical features of hypertensive encephalopathy: papilloedema, cerebral oedema or significant hypertension.[36] Because the enzyme nitric oxide synthase is a haemoprotein and nitric oxide is a major vascular dilator, the authors hypothesise that severe haem deficiency during acute porphyric attacks may cause unopposed cerebral vasoconstriction due to a decrease in cerebral nitric oxide production.

It is difficult to know whether Mr Cogan's comment on subject 1.9.2 was drawn from a contemporary textbook or reflected his experience with the Chester porphyria family. We can only speculate that some vascular phenomenon, presumably mediated by a humoral or neurogenic insult, caused the retinal haemorrhages – and perhaps the renal damage – in this subject, foreshadowing the subsequent hypertension. The occurrence and cause of the supposed angiospasm have attracted little interest in the literature until recently. As long ago as 1945 Denny-Brown and Sciarra[31] suggested the presence of some locally acting vasoconstrictor substance. It is hoped that the mouse model will provide some answers, in particular confirming or refuting the nitric oxide theory.

## Psychiatric morbidity

Ten porphyric subjects have received treatment at the County Mental Hospital and, as far as we know, no non-porphyric family members have needed psychiatric care (Chapter 11). At least four developed psychoses after barbiturate treatment, and one while receiving tricyclic antidepressants.

## Epilepsy

Epilepsy is relatively common at the peak of a porphyric crisis,[12,24,25] and may be related to hyponatraemia or hypertensive encephalopathy. The EEG is abnormal in the majority of patients experiencing an acute attack, and persists in some subjects during remission.[37]

*1.5.2*: admitted to Chester Royal Infirmary in 1964 at the age of 43 years. He was treated with phenobarbitone, and five days later became psychotic and had an epileptic fit. He was transferred to the County Mental Hospital and given further phenobarbitone as an aid to EEG interpretation – whereupon he developed a further confusional episode. Blood pressure readings and serum electrolytes are not available.

*1.5.5*: his brother, had a major seizure at the County Mental Hospital shortly before he developed meningism and coma from which he died, but necropsy failed to reveal the cause. At the time of the seizure, his blood pressure was 150/90 mmHg, and urea and electrolytes were normal (Chapter 6).

*1.6.3*: had major seizures during her long admission in 1954 at the age of 23 years, with complete paralysis complicating barbiturate treatment of malignant hypertension (Chapter 4). Her EEG was consistent with gross brain damage, and remained abnormal 12 months into remission.

*1.6.5*: her brother, was discharged from the Army in 1958, aged 20, because of epileptic fits (Chapter 6). He was treated with phenobarbitone, and developed abdominal pain and vomiting. Two months later he was admitted to Clatterbridge Hospital with a typical porphyric crisis. An EEG showed gross abnormality consistent with generalised brain damage. His blood pressure at this time was 170/140 mmHg and his blood urea 17 mmol/l.

*1.6.5.3*: daughter of 1.6.5, had an epileptic seizure during one of her 14 admissions at a time when her serum sodium was 115 mmol/l.

*1.9.3*: died of bulbar palsy in the 16th week of pregnancy, having had a major seizure the previous night. Her blood pressure and serum sodium level are not known.

*1.8.3.3*: had two seizures on one of her 17 admissions (Chapter 6) when her serum sodium was 114 mmol/l. At this time, her blood pressure was 220/120 mmHg and her pulse rate 140/min.

## Asthma, atopy and nasal polyps

Peter Dobson, the fisherman, was known to have asthma (his daughter (1.6) told her asthmatic daughter (1.6.6) that the affliction had come from grandfather Peter). Church[9] found that 10 porphyric members of the kindred had asthma, but no non-porphyric members. Moreover, two porphyric family members (1.1.5 (Chapter 5), 1.6.5) had porphyric crises after surgery for nasal polyps, a condition known to be associated with intrinsic non-allergic asthma. Two further members of generation III (1.6.1, 1.6.2) and two members of generation IV (1.1.1.1, 1.9.1.2) have nasal polyps. Church could not explain these findings, but pointed out that Meissner[38] had mentioned a possible association between porphyria and the inheritance of more than one other dominant trait. The atopy gene has subsequently been localised to chromosome 11q,[39] on which also lies the gene for Chester porphyria.[40,41] We extended the study of atopy prevalence in the Chester kindred, and have found no difference between those with and without porphyria (Chapter 10).

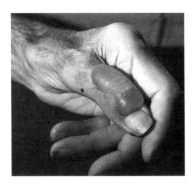

**Fig 1**. Bullous lesion on finger of subject 1.9.2.

## Dermatological features

Bekerus noted that her index case (1.1.5) had pustules on the face which led to scarring, although his sister (1.1.6) remembers this was ascribed to acne. McDonagh, with the benefit of a contemporary photograph, believes the lesion was most probably rosacea with an element of the lymphoedema often seen with chronic variants of this condition. This interpretation would also fit with Bekerus' history of photo-exacerbation. She mentions susceptibility to sunburn in a few other family members. We know of the following:

*1.6.5.3*: develops an urticarial reaction in strong sunlight, mainly on her lower legs and feet, which we have assumed to be solar urticaria.

*1.8.3.3*: the young woman who died of respiratory paralysis age 25 years (Chapter 6) had a swarthy hirsute appearance but there was no mention of photosensitivity.

*1.9.2*: developed bullous lesions on the distal fingers (Fig 1) after starting haemodialysis in the year of his death (Chapter 8, Part 4). He was not on frusemide, which has also been implicated.[42]

Despite the above, and having seen numerous family members over the years, none of whom have skin fragility on scratching with a finger-nail (Nikolsky's sign), we are unconvinced that any subject has had skin lesions of the type seen in porphyria variegata. Bullous lesions, akin to those of variegate porphyria, are well-known in patients receiving haemodialysis.[43,44] The bullous disease of haemodialysed patients may or may not be associated with increased levels of porphyrins.

## Discussion

The medical misfortunes of the scions of our family truly deserve the sobriquet *la petite simulatrice*. It took several decades to piece together the story because family members attended numerous different GPs in the city, and such was the miscellany of presentations that members were admitted as emergencies or referred to different specialists in any one of the four Chester hospitals (Table 1). Their abdominal pains were non-specific and attended by normal investigations, while the frequent psychiatric disturbance invited suspicions of hysteria. No one clinician's experience encompassed the premature deaths and prolonged hospital admissions experienced by some subjects, and it is not surprising that the consequent fear and despair turned, in some families and individuals, to resentment of the healing professions or denial that the taint afflicted their pedigree. Thus, in the family of eight siblings, 1.2.1–8, of whom

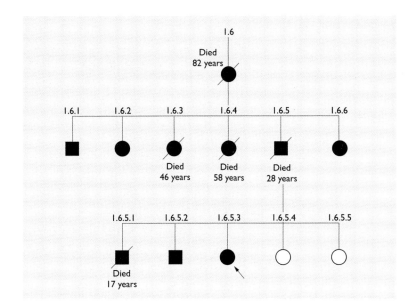

**Fig 2.** Family tree of Peter and Sarah Dobson's sixth child (arrow shows our index case 1.6.5.3)
○ = female;
□ = male;
●, ■ = symptomatic porphyria;
◖, ◪ = dead.

four brothers died of porphyria, none of the surviving four agreed to be tested by Bekerus and only one, 1.2.6, has been tested since and is positive.

The protean presentations of porphyria are illustrated by several families belonging to the Chester kindred. We have chosen the family of Peter Dobson's sixth child, 1.6, as an example (Fig 2). To date, she has had six children, 18 grandchildren, and five great-grandchildren:

*1.6*: wife of a storekeeper, died age 81 years in a psychogeriatric ward at the County Mental Hospital. She was not known to have had por-phyric symptoms, but had latent porphyria because she had raised urin-ary porphobilinogen and had porphyric children. She had hypertension, which is also regarded as a marker for porphyria in our kindred. We believe that five of her six children are porphyric.

*1.6.1*: an insurance agent, was born in 1926 and had repeated attacks of abdominal and back pain and headache from the late 1940s. He is currently well, but hypertensive. His porphyria biochemistry is positive. He was all too aware of the premature deaths of five young cousins (1.2.1, 1.2.3, 1.2.4, 1.2.8, 1.9.3), his brother (1.6.5) and sister (1.6.3), and so limited his family to one daughter.

*1.6.2*: born in 1927, has positive biochemistry but has never had por-phyric symptoms (ie she has latent porphyria).

*1.6.3*: wife of a gas fitter, died age 46 in 1978. She presented age 23 years with malignant hypertension, subsequently complicated by psychosis and flaccid paralysis (as described in Chapter 4). She died of cerebellar haemorrhage. Her porphyria biochemistry was positive.

103

```
                                    J. Rivers Esq.,
                                    Secretary,
                                    Service Department,
                                    British Legion,
                                    Pall Mall,
                                    London S.W.1


                      - 2 -

        When admitted to the Royal Naval Hospital, Chatham, he
    was diagnosed as cerebral dyarhythmia and his epileptiform
    blackouts were treated with phenobarbitone. He was transferred
    to the Royal Herbert Hospital, Woolwich, where further barbitirate
    treatment was given. On leaving Hospital the barbiturates were
    discontinued comnpletely. At this time, after leaving Hospital
    he had further attacke of abdominal pain, vomiting and diarrhoea.
    These were probably due to his porphyria and were possibly
    precipitated by the use of barbiturates. His acute attack which
    caused his admission to our Hospital occurred two months later
    and he had been off barbiturates for that period. There was no
    evidence that his treatment precipitated this acute attack.
```

**Fig 3**. Part of letter from Dr RR Hughes' medical registrar to the British Legion concerning subject 1.6.5 (1958).

*1.6.4*: wife of a storeman, born in 1932 and died in 1990, had latent porphyria (like her sister, 1.6.2).

*1.6.5*: an aircraft fitter, died age 37 in 1976. He had abdominal pain and an epileptic attack in the Army (Chapter 6). Biochemical tests for porphyria were positive (Fig 3). He had a porphyric crisis after nasal polypectomy, and died of malignant hypertension, cerebral haemorrhage and porphyria.

*1.6.6*: the youngest sibling, born in 1944, has negative biochemical tests for porphyria but has asthma.

Of 18 grandchildren of subject 1.6, six have positive biochemical tests for porphyria. As far as we know, only the children of 1.6.5 have had porphyric symptoms, and the other three grandchildren have latent porphyria (Fig 2).

*1.6.5.1*: died age 17 years in 1977 of bulbar palsy after presenting with abdominal pain (Chapter 6).

*1.6.5.3*: his sister, our index case, the schoolgirl who had 14 admissions with abdominal pain, sometimes complicated by paralysis.

*1.6.5.2*: their brother, has headaches, swollen optic discs probably due to drusen, but only one crisis with abdominal pain.

The family history explains the anguish of the mother of my index case (Chapter 1). Within six months she lost her husband (1.6.5) and eldest son (1.6.5.1), and one year later her husband's sister (1.6.3). These deaths presaged the 14 hospital admissions of her eldest daughter, 1.6.5.3, with severe porphyric crises, sometimes complicated by paralysis. The final dénouement was the referral to a physician (GRY) with a naïve understanding of the condition.

Several authors emphasise that the majority of subjects inheriting a gene for one of the acute hepatic porphyrias never experience symptoms. The percentage (75%) of porphyric subjects in generation III of our kindred with manifest symptoms (Table 2) is well above that reported in other series,[5,6,45,46] whereas the 40% with manifest symptoms in generation IV is almost identical to that of Kauppinen and Mustajoki's Finnish experience in 206 porphyric subjects.[7] An explanation of this twofold difference from one generation to the next can be found both in the environment and in medical practice.

*Environmental and medical factors*

*Barbiturates.* At least eight of our subjects' porphyric crises were associated with barbiturate administration in the era when these drugs were a panacea for many ills. The introduction of barbiturates coincided with an increase in the death rate in Northern Sweden (where porphyria is common), a phenomenon attributed by Waldenström[1] both to the increased use of barbiturates and evacuation of patients to secondary care centres where barbiturates were again used as sedatives or for surgery. Goldberg in 1959[12] and Ridley ten years later[24] both found 77% of their subjects with paralysis had received barbiturates.

Eales and Linder in 1962[14] found these drugs implicated in 47 of 107 (44%) attacks of variegate porphyria – indeed, Dean suggested in 1963[16] that variegate porphyria was virtually benign until unveiled by the introduction of barbiturates in 1903.

For these reasons, the acute porphyrias have been described as 'toxico-genetic diseases'.[47]

*Smoking.* Goldberg's group[48] has shown an association between cigarette smoking and the induction of repeated acute attacks of porphyria. Among their patients with symptomatic porphyria, 44% of smokers but only 11% of non-smokers had more than one attack. Paradoxically, the latent and symptomatic groups of patients with acute intermittent porphyria had almost identical proportions of smokers and non-smokers, suggesting that smoking is not the primary precipitant of acute attacks. We have shown (Chapter 10) that smoking is more prevalent in the porphyric than in the non-porphyric members of our family, but the sample size was small. This contrasts with smoking prevalence in the porphyria kindred in

Arjeplog, Sweden, where Andersson and Lithner[8] showed that both symptomatic and latent porphyria subjects smoke less than matched (but not family) controls. The symptomatic subjects smoked more than the latent porphyrics, but the difference was not statistically significant.

*Sunlight.* The high prevalence of acute porphyria in certain parts of the world has led to the suggestion that other environmental factors may play a role.[49] One such factor is sunlight, as found in South Africa.

*Lead toxicity.* Lead is known to interfere with pyrrole metabolism by inhibiting several enzymes of haem biosynthesis, including delta-aminolaevulinic acid dehydratase and ferrochelatase, thus causing increased levels of delta-aminolaevulinic acid and coproporphyrin in the urine and accumulation of protoporphyrin in erythrocytes.[15] Many of the clinical features of lead poisoning (eg abdominal colic, constipation, motor neuropathy) are also seen in acute attacks of hepatic porphyria. Most of the porphyric subjects in Swedish Lapland come from two valleys where there are some of the largest lead mines in the world.[49]

Until 1982, Chester had within its boundaries one of the largest lead smelting and manufacturing works in Great Britain, but lead levels in our patients have been normal, and their biochemical features do not correspond with classical lead poisoning. In 1843, at the age of 20, Samuel Dobson, Peter Dobson's great-uncle, was a seaman on board the flat (or sailing) barge *Patent*, which was owned by the Chester Leadworks and carried lead from Bagillt, Clwyd, to Liverpool, returning with imported ore. Chester's association with lead has an even earlier provenance: a lead ingot found on the site of the gas works has an inscription dating it to AD 74.[50]

*Alcohol.* A difference in alcohol consumption between generations III and IV of our family might explain the different expression of symptomatic porphyria. This has not been surveyed, and we know of only one subject (1.8.1) whose porphyric crises followed heavy drinking. Kauppinen and Mustajoki[7] in their survey of 206 porphyric subjects found 40% reported post-alcohol symptoms suggestive of porphyria, in most cases occasional and mild. Two subjects had repeated episodes of motor neuropathy associated with heavy drinking.

### Latency

The reason why the majority of carriers of the porphyria gene remain latent is not known. A number of studies have assessed methods of detecting latent cases in affected families.[5,6,45,46] Urine analysis is of limited value because increased excretion of delta-aminolaevulinic acid and porphobilinogen is present in only one in every three latent cases,[51] and there is considerable overlap in blood porphobilinogen deaminase levels between normal and porphyric subjects.[5,6] Many subjects with high urinary excretion of porphobilinogen remain asymptomatic, but Kauppinen and Mustajoki[7] believe that non-excretors of porphobilinogen have a good chance of remaining asymptomatic: 15 of their subjects with porphyria and normal porphobilinogen excretion remained asymptomatic during follow-up. This suggests that non-excretors of porphobilinogen are at lower risk and might, for example, be allowed to take sex hormone medication under supervision (Chapter 4).

We have shown above that symptomatic, as opposed to latent, porphyria is unusually common in our pedigree compared with published series from elsewhere. The Chester kindred differs in a further respect, in that males rather than females are more likely to be symptomatic (Table 2), contrary to Moore *et al*'s summary[15] that:

> *all major series show a female preponderance of symptomatic though not latent disease.*

Voswinckel[52] and Rimington[53] make a persuasive case that Hippocrates described a case of acute porphyria. His patient displayed disorientation, intermittent convulsions, with severe and continuous pains, then she became comatose and, finally, unrestrained with the passage of dark urine. On the third day, copious menstruation occurred. As so often happens in the study of the history of medicine, the writings of Hippocrates foreshadow modern-day endeavours, although it defies conventional explanation how he amassed such a fascinating cornucopia of diseases in what must have been a small catchment population.

# References

1 Waldenström J. Neurological symptoms caused by so called acute porphyria. *Acta Psychiatrica et Neurologica* 1939; **14**: 375–9.

2 Gajdos A, Gajdos-Török M. Studies on the porphyrias in France. *South African Journal of Laboratory and Clinical Medicine* 1963; **9**: 295–300.

3 Goldberg A, Rimington C. *Diseases of porphyrin metabolism*. Springfield, IL: Charles C Thomas, 1962.

4 Jones R, Lydeard S. Irritable bowel syndrome in the general population. *British Medical Journal* 1992; **304**: 87–90.

5 Lamon JM, Frykholm BC, Tschudy DP. Family evaluations in acute intermittent porphyria using red cell uroporphyrinogen 1 synthetase. *Journal of Medical Genetics* 1979; **16**: 134–9.

6  McColl KEL, Moore MR, Thompson GG, Goldberg A. Screening for latent acute intermittent porphyria: the value of measuring both leucocyte δ-aminolaevulinic acid synthase and erythrocyte uroporphyrinogen-l-synthase activities. *Journal of Medical Genetics* 1982; **19**: 271–6.

7  Kauppinen R, Mustajoki P. Prognosis of acute porphyria: occurrence of acute attacks, precipitating factors, and associated diseases. *Medicine* 1992; **71**: 1–13.

8  Andersson C, Lithner F. Hypertension and renal disease in patients with acute intermittent porphyria. *Journal of Internal Medicine* 1994; **236**: 169–75.

9  Church SE. The Chester porphyria. MD Thesis, University of Liverpool, 1986.

10  Church SE, McColl KE, Moore MR, Youngs GR. Hypertension and renal impairment as complications of acute porphyria. *Nephrology Dialysis Transplantation* 1992; **7**: 986–90.

11  Waldenström J. The porphyrias as inborn errors of metabolism. *American Journal of Medicine* 1957; **22**: 758–73.

12  Goldberg A. Acute intermittent porphyria: a study of 50 cases. *Quarterly Journal of Medicine* 1959; NS **28**: 183–209.

13  Markovitz M. Acute intermittent porphyria: a report of five cases and a review of the literature. *Annals of Internal Medicine* 1954; **41**: 1170–88.

14  Eales L, Linder GC. Porphyria – the acute attack: an analysis of 80 cases. *South African Medical Journal* 1962; **36**: 284–92.

15  Moore MR, McColl KEL, Rimington C, Goldberg A. *Disorders of porphyrin metabolism*. New York: Plenum, 1987.

16  Dean G. *The porphyrias: a story of inheritance and environment*. London: Pitman, 1963.

17  Dover SB, Plenderleith L, Moore MR, McColl KE. Safety of general anaesthesia and surgery in acute hepatic porphyria. *Gut* 1994; **35**: 1112–5.

18  Meissner PN, Harrison GG, Hift RJ. Propofol as an I.V. anaesthetic induction agent in variegate porphyria. *British Journal of Anaesthesia* 1991; **66**: 60–5.

19  Eales L, Day RS, Blekkenhorst GH. The clinical and biochemical features of variegate porphyria: an analysis of 300 cases studied at Groote Schuur Hospital, Capetown. *International Journal of Biochemistry* 1980; **12**: 837–53.

20  Chaudhary NA, Truelove SC. The irritable colon syndrome. A study of the clinical features, predisposing causes, and prognosis in 130 cases. *Quarterly Journal of Medicine* NS 1962; **31**: 307–22.

21  Kasich AM, Rafsky JC. Clinical evaluation of an anticholinergic in the irritable colon syndrome. A double blind study of tricyclamol. *American Journal of Gastroenterology* 1959; **31**: 47–52.

22  *British National Formulary*. London: British Medical Association and the Royal Pharmaceutical Society, 1995.

23  Lip GYH, McColl KEL, Goldberg A, Moore MR. Smoking and recurrent attacks of acute intermittent porphyria. *British Medical Journal* 1991; **302**: 507.

24  Ridley A. The neuropathy of acute intermittent porphyria. *Quarterly Journal of Medicine* NS 1969; **38**: 307–33.

25  Bonkowsky HL, Schady W. Neurologic manifestations of acute porphyria. *Seminars in Liver Disease* 1982; **2**: 108–24.

26  Puy H, Deybach J-C, Bogdan A, Callebert J, *et al.* Increased δ-aminolevulinic acid and decreased pineal melatonin production. A common event in acute porphyria studies in the rat. *Journal of Clinical Investigation* 1996; **97**: 104–10.

27  Lindberg RLP, Porcher C, Grandchamp B, Ledermann B, *et al.* Porphobilinogen deaminase deficiency in mice causes a neuropathy resembling that of human hepatic porphyria (letter). *Nature Genetics* 1996; **12**: 195–9.

28  Wetterberg L. *A neuropsychiatric and genetical investigation of acute intermittent porphyria*. Stockholm: Svenska Bokforlaget, 1976.

29  Sze G. Cortical brain lesions in acute intermittent porphyria (letter). *Annals of Internal Medicine* 1996; **125**: 422–3.

30  Yeung Laiwah AAC, Mactier R, McColl KEL, Moore MR, Goldberg A. Early onset chronic renal failure as a complication of acute intermittent porphyria. *Quarterly Journal of Medicine* 1983; **205**: 92–8.

31  Denny-Brown D, Sciarra D. Changes in the nervous system in acute porphyria. *Brain* 1945; **68**: 1–16.

32  Wolter JR, Clark RL, Kallet HA. Ocular involvement in acute intermittent porphyria. *American Journal of Ophthalmology* 1972; **74**: 666–74.

33  DeFrancisco M, Savino PJ, Schatz NJ. Optic atrophy in acute intermittent porphyria. *American Journal of Ophthalmology* 1979; **87**: 221–4.

34  Barnes HD, Boshoff PH. Ocular lesions in patients with porphyria. *American Medical Association Archives of Ophthalmology* 1952; **48**: 567–80.

35  Kupferschmidt H, Bont A, Schnorf H, Landis T, *et al.* Transient cortical blindness and biooccipital brain lesions in two patients with acute intermittent porphyria. *Annals of Internal Medicine* 1995; **123**: 598–600.

36  Kupferschmidt H, Meier PJ (letter). Cortical brain lesions in acute intermittent porphyria. *Annals of Internal Medicine* 1996; **125**: 423.

37  Albers JW, Robertson WC, Daube JR. Electrodiagnostic findings in acute porphyric neuropathy. *Muscle and Nerve* 1978; **1**: 292–6.

38  Meissner DM. Porphyria in the Afrikaner population (letter). *South African Medical Journal* 1984; **65**: 277.

39  Cookson WO, Sharp PA, Faux JA, Hopkin JM. Linkage between immunoglobulin E responses underlying asthma and rhinitis and chromosome 11q. *Lancet* 1989; **i**: 1292–4.

40  Norton B. *A genetic study of Chester porphyria*. MD Thesis, University of Liverpool, 1993.

41 Norton B, Lanyon WG, Moore MR, Porteous M, *et al*. Evidence for involvement of a second genetic locus on chromosome 11q in porphyrin metabolism. *Human Genetics* 1993; **91**: 576–8.

42 Shelley WB, Shelley ED. Blisters of the fingertips: a variant of bullous dermatosis of hemodialysis. *Journal of the American Academy of Dermatology* 1989; **21**: 1049–51.

43 Gilchrest B, Rowe JW, Mihm MC. Bullous dermatosis of haemodialysis. *Annals of Internal Medicine* 1975; **83**: 480–3.

44 Mascaro JM, Herrero C, Lecha M, Muniesa AM. Uroporphyrinogen-decarboxylase deficiencies: porphyria cutanea tarda and related conditions. *Seminars in Dermatology* 1986; **5**: 115–24.

45 Bottomley SS, Bonkowsky HL, Kreimer-Birnbaum M. The diagnosis of acute intermittent porphyria. Usefulness and limitations of the erythrocyte uroporphyrinogen I synthase assay. *American Journal of Clinical Pathology* 1981; **76**: 133–9.

46 Pierach CA, Weimer MK, Cardinal RA, Bossenmaier IC, Blommer JR. Red blood cell porphobilinogen deaminase in the evaluation of acute intermittent porphyria. *Journal of the American Medical Association* 1987; **257**: 60–1.

47 Moore MR, Hift RJ. Drugs in the acute porphyrias – toxicogenetic diseases. *Cellular and Molecular Biology* 1997: **43**: 89–94.

48 Lip GYH, McColl KEL, Goldberg A, Moore MR. Smoking and recurrent attacks of acute intermittent porphyria. *British Medical Journal* 1991; **302**: 507.

49 Waldenström J, Haeger-Aronsen B. The porphyrias: a genetic problem. In: Steinberg AG, Bearn AG (eds). *Progress in medical genetics*, vol V. London: Grune and Stratton, 1967: 58–101.

50 Thompson FH. *Deva – Roman Chester*. Chester: Grosvenor Museum, 1959.

51 Grelier M, Grandchamp B, Phung N, de Verneuil H, *et al*. Détection de la porphyrie aiguë intermittente par le dosage de l'urosynthétase. *La Nouvelle Presse Médicale* 1977; **6**: 1045–7.

52 Voswinckel P. A constant source of surprises: acute porphyria. Two cases reported by Hippocrates and Sigmund Freud. *History of Psychiatry* 1990; **1**: 159–68.

53 Rimington C. Was Hippocrates the first to describe a case of acute porphyria? *International Journal of Biochemistry* 1993; **25**: 1351–2.

*Part 3*

# The ramifications of
# porphyria explored

*Chapter 8*

# Hypertension and chronic renal failure as complications of acute porphyria

SUSAN CHURCH AND GILES YOUNGS

## Preamble

Early in our investigation of the Chester porphyria we became aware of the high prevalence of hypertension and chronic renal failure,[1] and in 1985 performed a formal retrospective and prospective study (published as an MD thesis in 1986[2] and in *Nephrology Dialysis Transplantation* in 1992[3]). The survey was repeated in 1995 as part of our asthma and atopy study (Chapter 10), and consideration was given to amalgamating the findings with those of 1985 into one report. On reflection, this would have been difficult for two reasons:

- Three porphyric grandchildren have died since 1985, and it would be inappropriate to use blood pressure and renal function data taken 10 years apart as one statistical whole.
- The two populations attending were dissimilar, the 52 subjects examined in 1985 came only from generations III and IV, while in the later survey 21 of the 57 examined came from generation V. Most of these great-great-grandchildren were under 20 years of age, suitable for atopy testing but unlikely to have developed hypertension or renal failure.

The 1985 study is therefore reproduced verbatim (with kind permission of the publishers) as Part 1 of this chapter, with the 1995 study given in Part 2. These data, and the implications of two subsequently published studies,[4,5] are analysed in Part 3, with special reference to the role of gender and porphyria activity in the risk of subsequent development of hypertension and renal failure. The case

113

histories of the grandchildren in the Chester family with hypertension and renal impairment are presented in Part 4. Family members with hypertension or renal failure are listed in Table 3.

## Part 1: Hypertension and renal impairment as complications of acute porphyria*

*SE Church, KEL McColl, MR Moore and GR Youngs*

Hypertension and uraemia are commonly seen in the acute crisis of acute intermittent[6] and variegate porphyria.[7] That these complications may persist has been the subject of only two reports.[8,9] Latent porphyric subjects (who have inherited the enzyme defect but have never had symptoms of acute porphyria) have not been studied before.

We studied a large family with acute porphyria living in Chester. Affected members present with acute attacks resembling those seen in acute intermittent porphyria.[1] This form is biochemically unusual in that a dual enzyme deficiency is present.[10] Each affected subject has reduced activity of both porphobilinogen (PBG) deaminase and protoporphyrinogen oxidase, giving an excretion pattern that resembles either acute intermittent or variegate porphyria, and some have an intermediate pattern.

Members of the Chester kindred have a high incidence of premature death associated with hypertension and renal failure. We have studied the relationship between porphyric status and the incidence of hypertension and renal impairment in living members of the family who have overt and latent porphyria, and in those who are normal.

### Subjects and methods

The family has produced 200 descendants who still live in Chester.[1] There is no known consanguinity. This study is divided into two parts:

*(a) Prospective study of 52 living members of generations III and IV*

Porphyric status, blood pressure and renal function were determined during remission. Classification of porphyric status was determined by the activities of PBG deaminase, protoporphyrinogen

*Reprinted, with kind permission of the publishers, from an article in *Nephrology Dialysis Transplantation*.[3]

Minor editorial changes have been made in accordance with the Royal College of Physicians' house style. References, Tables and Figures have been renumbered consecutively through the chapter.

oxidase and delta-aminolaevulinic acid synthase in peripheral blood cells together with quantitative analysis of urinary and faecal excretion.[10]

Hypertension was defined as a systolic pressure of 160 mmHg or above and a diastolic pressure of 100 mmHg or above (Korotkoff, phase 5) obtained with a standard mercury sphygmomanometer and stethoscope with readings to ±2 mmHg.[11] The patients were resting lying, and the mean of two recordings were noted. An attempt was made to reduce any variability such as the time of day and degree of stress. In many cases the patients, having refused to attend hospital, had their assessments made at home in a quiet environment. All blood pressures were recorded by one observer (SEC) blinded regarding the presence or absence of a biochemical defect in three-quarters of the patients examined, since initially the porphyric status was only known in seven patients who had suffered acute attacks and in one patient who also had renal impairment. Three patients were on antihypertensive treatment prior to entering the survey, and the ages and levels at which hypertension was first noted are those used in the analysis.

Renal function was assessed by the measurement of plasma creatinine (normal ranges 75–120 nmol/l in males and 60–115 nmol/l in females) and creatinine clearance (normal ranges 80–125 ml/min in males and 70–115 ml/min in females). The age at which renal impairment was first noted was that used in the statistical analysis. At the time of the study no patients were on dialysis or had received a kidney transplant.

Results were analysed by Student's $t$-test. Creatinine and creatinine clearance have a skew distribution and thus required logarithmic transformation prior to analysis.

*(b) Retrospective analysis of the causes of death in generations II and III*

All information regarding the causes of death and preceding illnesses was obtained from patients' case records and death certification. This included all 10 siblings from generation II and 17 siblings (of 38) in generation III.

## Results

*(a) Prospective study*

Twenty-six (12 male) of the 52 family members examined had porphyria and 26 (11 male) did not. There was no significant difference between the mean age of the porphyric (mean 36 years, range 19–57) and non-porphyric subjects (mean 35 years, range 17–58).

115

**Table 1.** Differences in blood pressure between porphyric and non-porphyric subjects and between porphyric subjects according to clinical and biochemical status.

| | No. | Mean age (years) (range) | Mean blood pressure (mmHg) | |
| --- | --- | --- | --- | --- |
| | | | Systolic (range) | Diastolic (range) |
| Non-porphyric subjects | 23 | 35 (17–56) | 123 (100–160) | 74 (60–90) |
| All porphyric subjects | 24 | 36 (19–57) | *141 (110–200) | *88 (60–120) |
| *Porphyric subjects:* | | | | |
| symptomatic | 7 | 41 (22–50) | *148 (110–200) | *91 (60–110) |
| latent | 17 | 34 (19–57) | *138 (110–190) | *86 (65–120) |
| *Porphyric subjects:* | | | | |
| increased excretion of haem precursors | 16 | 38 (20–57) | 145 (110–200) | 91 (60–120) |
| normal excretion of haem precursors | 8 | 33 (19–54) | 133 (110–170) | 82 (65–100) |

* Significantly higher than non-porphyric subjects with $p < 0.05$.

Of the 26 porphyric subjects studied, seven had experienced clinical attacks of acute porphyria and 18 had increased excretion of haem precursors.

Systolic and diastolic blood pressures were significantly greater in the porphyric than in the non-porphyric subjects ($p < 0.05$) (Table 1). Eight of the 24 (33%) porphyric subjects studied were hypertensive compared with only one of the 23 (4%) non-porphyric subjects (Fig 1). The prevalence of hypertension was increased both in porphyric subjects with previous attacks (3 of 7) and in those who were clinically latent (5 of 17) when each was compared alone with the non-porphyric subjects.

Plasma creatinine was significantly greater in the porphyric than in the non-porphyric subjects ($p < 0.02$) (Table 2; Fig 1). The creatinine clearances were significantly less in the porphyric subjects who had suffered acute attacks than in those who were clinically latent ($p < 0.05$) (Table 2). Creatinine clearances were reduced in nine of 23 (39%) porphyric and three of 17 (18%) non-porphyric subjects, but this difference did not reach statistical significance ($0.05 < p < 0.1$). Those with reduced creatinine clearance showed no evidence of increased urinary protein excretion or casts. Intravenous urograms and renal isotope scans were performed in subjects with impaired renal function whenever the subject was agreeable. Intravenous urograms were normal in four of the porphyric subjects, and two (1 overt and 1 latent) porphyric subjects had bilateral small kidneys. Renal isotope scans in six such porphyric subjects showed a reduced mean effective renal plasma

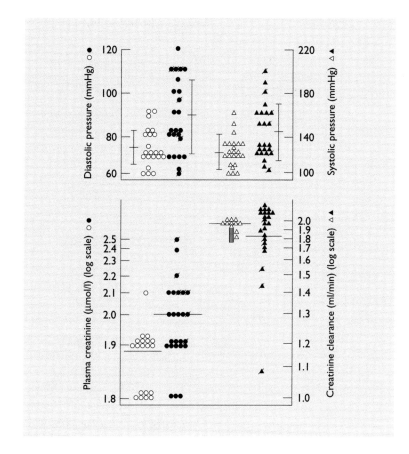

Fig 1. Individual blood pressure and renal function values for the living porphyric and non-porphyric family members (horizontal line (upper graph): mean blood pressure; horizontal line (lower graph): geometric mean for the creatinine data; vertical line ±1 standard deviation).
○,△ = non-porphyric patients.
Porphyric patients:
●, ▲ = latent;
◗,◭ = previous acute attacks.

Table 2. Differences in renal function between porphyric and non-porphyric subjects and between porphyric subjects according to clinical and biochemical status.

| | No. | Mean age (years) (range) | Geometric mean plasma creatinine (μmol/l)(range) | No. | Mean age (years) (range) | Geometric mean creatinine clearance (ml/min)(range) |
|---|---|---|---|---|---|---|
| Non-porphyric subjects | 24 | 35 (17–56) | 79 (63–115) | 17 | 32 (17–56) | 94 (70–126) |
| All porphyric subjects | 25 | 36 (19–57) | *99 (64–330) | 23 | 35 (19–57) | 74 (12–151) |
| *Porphyric subjects:* | | | | | | |
| symptomatic | 7 | 41 (22–50) | *132 (74–330) | 7 | 41 (22–50) | *50 (12–100) |
| latent | 18 | 34 (19–57) | 87 (64–243) | 16 | 33 (19–57) | 85 (27–152) |
| *Porphyric subjects:* | | | | | | |
| increased excretion of haem precursors | 18 | 36 (20–57) | 107 (65–330) | 16 | 37 (22–57) | 68 (12–152) |
| normal excretion of haem precursors | 7 | 30 (19–42) | 81 (64–139) | 7 | 30 (19–42) | 87 (54–123) |

* Significantly higher/lower than non-porphyric subjects with $p < 0.02$.

flow of 312 ml/min per 1.73 m² (range 145–412) (normal range 544–680 ml/min per 1.73 m²).

There was no significant difference in blood pressure, creatinine or creatinine clearance between those with porphyrin overproduction and those who had normal porphyrin excretion.

Of the five porphyric subjects who have both hypertension and renal impairment, only three have suffered clinical attacks of porphyria, and only one of these three was hypertensive during attacks. Of the three porphyric subjects who have hypertension but normal renal function, none has experienced a porphyric attack, and of the two with renal impairment and normal blood pressure only one has experienced an attack.

### (b) Retrospective survey

In generation II, where all 10 siblings are dead, few medical records are available for the study. However, of the six porphyric siblings, four are known to have had hypertension or renal failure.

Of the 38 grandchildren in generation III (19 porphyric) 17 are now dead and nine of these deaths were in known porphyric subjects. Five of the porphyric deaths (2 male and 3 female; mean age 47 years) were directly related to hypertension, and three had additional renal impairment. Three of these patients had previously suffered acute attacks and one of them had documented hypertension in one of these attacks. Of the eight deaths in the non-porphyric subjects, or any of unknown status in generation III, none was attributable to hypertension or renal impairment.

### (c) Combined retrospective and prospective data of generation III

The 38 grandchildren in generation III can be considered as a whole by combining the results of the retrospective and prospective studies. Ten (5 living) of 16 (62%) porphyric patients whose blood pressures have been measured were hypertensive. Seven (4 living) of 14 (50%) porphyric patients had renal impairment and all of these patients were hypertensive.

Renal tissue was obtained from three of these subjects (2 at post-mortem) and all showed extensive loss of renal tissue with evidence of nephrosclerosis with no underlying identifying features.

Of the 21 grandchildren suspected not to suffer from porphyria, none had hypertension or renal impairment.

### Discussion

This study reveals that patients with porphyria suffer from chronic hypertension and impaired renal function when compared with the non-porphyric members of the Chester family. There has been one previous report that survivors of attacks of acute intermittent porphyria may develop chronic hypertension[8] and one report of early-onset renal impairment.[9] The former study found hypertension in 42% of patients still alive 20 years after presenting with acute porphyric crises. Of six patients who had died, hypertension was implicated in three deaths. In the latter study, six of 65 (9%) of unrelated porphyric subjects in remission had early-onset chronic renal failure leading to death in four. This association between acute porphyria, hypertension and chronic renal impairment, with death from cardiovascular disease, is supported by the retrospective data obtained from our study.

This study enabled a prospective comparison to be made between porphyric and non-porphyric subjects with a common genotype and phenotype. There was a significant difference in both diastolic and systolic blood pressures between porphyric and non-porphyric family members who were matched for age and sex. Combined population surveys suggest that 7% of the general population below 65 years of age have a diastolic blood pressure above 100 mmHg with 10–15% above 95 mmHg.[12] In contrast, we found that 33% of our living porphyric subjects below the age of 65 years had hypertension. Most importantly, latent porphyric subjects appeared to have the same risk as those who had previously had acute attacks.

The mechanism underlying the hypertension and renal impairment is not known. Transient hypertension complicates 30–50% of acute porphyric attacks.[6,7] It is ascribed to various aetiologies including adrenergic dysfunction, increased catecholamine excretion, and interruption of the baroreceptor reflex due to damaged vagal and glossopharyngeal nerves[13] analogous to the hypertension of the Guillain-Barré syndrome,[14] and acute paralytic poliomyelitis, which is sustained in 25% of cases.[15] The pressure lability itself, with episodically high levels in the acute attack, may result in vascular changes which may progress to irreversible hypertension. In patients who have died of poliomyelitis[15] and acute intermittent porphyria,[16] structural damage to the hypothalamus and brain stem nuclei has been described. Damage in these areas causes specific changes in baroreceptor function capable of producing more sustained hypertension.[17] However, in our living subjects, only four of the eight with hypertension have had clinical attacks of acute porphyria, and only one of these four is known to have been hypertensive during the attacks. Thus complications of the acute attacks such as neuropathy, oliguria or dehydration cannot fully explain the later development of hypertension and renal impairment.

Neuropathic changes, however, have been found in latent cases of porphyria.[18] These may be due to recurrent subclinical attacks of acute porphyria, the cumulative effect of which may result in permanent neuropathy with disruption of the baroreceptor reflex and lead to hypertension.

Progressive renal damage in most patients with hypertension is relatively slow and renal failure uncommon except with malignant hypertension. Thus the finding of renal impairment in some latent porphyric subjects, as well as those in remission, many of whom now have only mild or well-controlled hypertension or who are normotensive, suggests that the renal lesion may be primary. Renal tubular damage in subjects dying in porphyric crisis has been described in acute intermittent porphyria[19] and variegate porphyria.[20] It is suggested that excess porphyrins or their precursors are nephrotoxic, especially as the kidneys are now known to be partially responsible for porphyrin synthesis.[21,22] A common final pathway in the generation of secondary hypertension due to renal disease may be shared with lead toxicity which is also associated with hypertension in various studies.[23] It also remains possible that porphyria and hypertension are independent diseases but genetically linked. That the findings of hypertension and renal impairment in this family are related to the uniqueness of their dual enzyme deficiency is refuted by the few previous reports[8,9] of chronic hypertension and early-onset renal impairment in acute intermittent porphyria.

The investigation of the cause and full extent of the hypertension and renal impairment in this family was dogged by the non-attendance and poor compliance of these patients, both of which are typical of the porphyric personality. Despite this, the results presented are highly significant.

Hypertension and renal impairment have been the cause of considerable morbidity and mortality in the Chester kindred and these complications of porphyria are not recognised. Patients who have suffered attacks of porphyria should have their blood pressure and their renal function checked at regular intervals. In addition, our findings indicate that carriers of the porphyric trait who have never experienced an attack should also be monitored. For every one symptomatic porphyric patient there are 10 asymptomatic carriers.[24] The latter will therefore form the major workload of such a screening programme for detecting early hypertension and renal impairment related to porphyria. However, it is hoped that with effective treatment the marked increase in morbidity and mortality can be avoided.

## Part 2: 1995 survey of blood pressure and renal function in generations III, IV and V of the Chester porphyria family

In 1995 we wrote to 75 adult members of the family listed in our porphyria index, inviting them to attend the Countess of Chester Hospital with their children aged over seven years for lung function and atopy testing (described in Chapter 10). Blood pressure was recorded, and blood taken in each subject for measurement of urea and creatinine at the beginning and end of the session, as previously described. Nine of the 17 surviving members of generation III, 31 of generation IV, and 21 of generation V attended. There was no hypertension or renal impairment in the members of generation V. Five of six (83%) porphyric grandchildren and three of 12 (25%) porphyric great-grandchildren had hypertension, renal impairment or both. None of the 22 porphyria-negative subjects was affected. Table 3 combines the data from the 1985 and 1995 studies, and lists family members in generations II–IV with hypertension or renal failure. Overall, the morbidity and mortality due to hypertension and renal failure are shown for 13 of 24 (54%) porphyric members of generation III, and at least 7 of the 25 (28%) porphyric members of generation IV (not all 25 have had blood pressure and renal function measured).

The 1995 study by itself is of limited statistical value as the subjects tested are only a small sample of the population at risk, but the results are in agreement with the 1985 findings. The Chester experience is compared with that in Scotland, Finland and Sweden in Part 3.

## Part 3: Hypertension and renal failure in porphyria: the Chester experience compared with that in Scotland, Finland and Sweden

Since publication of our article in 1992,[3] two useful reports assessing the prevalence of hypertension and chronic renal failure in porphyria have appeared:

- a retrospective and prospective study of 268 Finnish subjects with porphyria by Kauppinen and Mustajoki in 1992,[4] and
- a case-control study of 50 Swedish subjects by Andersson and Lithner in 1994.[5]

**Table 3.** Hypertension and renal failure in members of generations II, III and IV

| Family notation | Sex | Por-phyria status | Age (years) at: | | Morbidity | Death certificate |
|---|---|---|---|---|---|---|
| | | | Diagnosis | Death | | |
| *Generation II* | | | | | | |
| 1.2 | M | U | U | 62 | | HT |
| 1.3 | F | U | U | 48 | | HT, RF |
| 1.4 | F | L | U | 59 | HT | CVA |
| 1.5 | M | S | U | 83 | HT | RF |
| 1.6 | F | L | U | 81 | HT | Pneumonia |
| *Generation III* | | | | | | |
| 1.1.1 | F | L | U | 63 | | HT, CVA |
| 1.1.5 | M | S | U | 40 | HT, RF | HT, RF |
| 1.1.6 | F | L | 35 | A | HT, RF | |
| 1.2.1 | M | S | U | 29 | | RF, Nephritis |
| 1.2.8 | M | S | U | 18 | | MHT |
| 1.4.1 | M | L | 50 | A | HT, RF | |
| 1.6.1* | M | S | U | A | HT | |
| 1.6.3 | F | S | 23 | 46 | MHT, RF | CVA |
| 1.6.5 | M | S | 37 | 37 | | MHT, CVA |
| 1.8.1 | M | S | 35 | A | HT, RF | |
| 1.8.2 | M | S | 49 | A | HT, RF | |
| 1.8.3 | F | S | 47 | 47 | HT, RF | RF |
| 1.9.2† | M | S | 45 | 55 | HT, RF | HT, RF, CVA |
| *Generation IV* | | | | | | |
| 1.1.1.1* | F | S | 46 | A | HT, RF | |
| 1.1.1.2 | M | L | 37 | A | RF | |
| 1.5.3.1 | M | S | 40 | A | HT | |
| 1.5.3.2 | F | L | 30 | A | HT | |
| 1.5.3.3 | F | S | 38 | A | HT | |
| 1.6.5.3‡ | F | S | 30 | A | RF | |
| 1.8.3.7 | M | S | 36 | A | HT, RF | |

\* developed HT since 1985 study
† died since 1985 study
‡ developed RF since 1985

A = alive
CVA = cerebrovascular accident
HT = hypertension
L = latent
MHT = malignant hypertension
RF = renal failure
S = symptomatic
U = unknown

## The Finnish study[4]

Kauppinen and Mustajoki studied 195 subjects with acute intermittent porphyria and 73 with variegate porphyria. Five of 96 (5%) deceased subjects, all women, died from chronic renal failure (chronic nephritis 2, glomerulonephritis 1, acute tubular necrosis 1, not stated 1), at a mean age of 54 years. There is no mention of hypertension as a cause of death. The prospective survey was drawn from questionnaires completed by 158 subjects. Thirty-eight (24%) had current or previous hypertension, and the occurrence was equal in those with symptomatic or latent porphyria. The age-specific prevalence rate of hypertension was higher than in the general population. Nine of the 158 (6%) reported renal failure, associated with hypertension in seven. Renal biopsies showed mesangial glomerulonephritis in one subject, and tubular fibrosis in another. The authors conclude that there is *probably* an increased incidence of hypertension and chronic renal failure in the subjects with acute porphyria.

## The Swedish study[5]

Andersson and Lithner surveyed, both retrospectively and prospectively, the prevalence of hypertension and renal failure in porphyric people in a municipality in Northern Sweden where the prevalence of porphyria is 2%. All patients tested had the same mutation in the PBG deaminase gene identifying the 'Norrland' family. During the study period, 33 subjects with porphyria had died, three (9%) from uraemia (chronic glomerulonephritis, chronic pyelonephritis and urinary tract obstruction). This contrasted with a 1% prevalence of death due to uraemia in a control group (odds ratio 9.4). Sixteen of the 33 (48%) deceased porphyric subjects had hypertension, 13 of the 19 (68%) with symptomatic porphyria and three of the 14 (21%) with latent porphyria (odds ratio, hypertension in deceased porphyrics compared with deceased controls, 7.9).

In the prospective study, 50 subjects with porphyria (25 symptomatic, 25 latent) were compared with 171 age-, gender- and domicile-matched controls. Overall, there was no difference in creatinine levels between the two groups, although a subgroup of eight women with symptomatic porphyria had significantly higher creatinine levels than their 26 controls. Hypertension was defined as a condition treated with hypertensive drugs. The prevalence in the control group was surprisingly high (52 of 171 (30%) subjects). Nevertheless, the prevalence of hypertension in the subjects with symptomatic porphyria (14 of 28 (50%)), was significantly higher than in controls (28 of 84 (33%)) and in those with latent porphyria (4 of 24 (17%)). The *actual* blood pressure readings were similar in all groups, but of course many of these subjects were receiving medication for hypertension.

## Comparison of five published studies of the prevalence of hypertension and renal failure in porphyria

The data from five studies of hypertension and renal impairment in porphyria are summarised in Table 4. Some conclusions are easily drawn, others are more tentative. The publications from Chester[2,3] and Sweden[5] both involved pedigrees with a defined genetic mutation, whereas the Finnish[4] and probably the Scottish[8,9] porphyric subjects were genetically diverse. The prospective Chester study compared blood pressure and renal function in porphyric subjects compared with their non-porphyric siblings and cousins, the Finnish subjects were compared with the general population, while the Swedish study used age- and gender-matched controls from the same municipality.

## Hypertension and renal failure in symptomatic versus latent porphyria

Two of the three prospective studies (Chester and Finland) found an increased prevalence of hypertension in both symptomatic and latent porphyria, whereas the Swedish study showed hypertension to be more common only in symptomatic subjects. Interpretation of the Swedish data is made difficult by the high prevalence (30%) of hypertension in the control group. It is difficult to say – and is not discussed by the authors – whether this reflects a high prevalence of hypertension in the municipality or a low threshold of treatment. Three of four retrospective studies (Scotland, Chester and Sweden) reported increased prevalence of hypertension in porphyria subjects, but no information was given in the Finnish study. In Chester, three deceased subjects (1.4, 1.6, 1.1.1) with latent porphyria had hypertension (Table 3) .

The Chester prospective study showed that renal impairment is found both in symptomatic and in latent porphyria subjects (Tables 2 and 3), but is statistically different from controls only in the former. Similarly in Sweden, reduced renal function is seen in both groups, but is significantly different from controls only in women with symptomatic porphyria. The renal impairment in Finnish subjects is not subdivided into symptomatic and latent

**Table 4.** Prevalence of hypertension and renal impairment in porphyric subjects in Scotland, Chester, Finland and Sweden

| | Scotland | | | | Chester | | Finland | | Sweden | |
|---|---|---|---|---|---|---|---|---|---|---|
| | 1975[8] | | 1983[9] | | 1986[2] & 1992[3] | | 1992[4] | | 1994[5] | |
| Expression of porphyria | S | L | S | L | S | L | S | L | S | L |
| *Hypertension:* | | | | | | | | | | |
| retrospective | Y | NT | NT | NT | Y | Y | NT | NT | Y | U |
| prospective | NT | NT | NT | NT | Y | Y | Y | Y | Y | NT |
| *Renal failure:* | | | | | | | | | | |
| retrospective | NT | NT | Y | NT | Y | NT | Y* | | Y | |
| prospective | NT | NT | NT | NT | Y | U | Y | | Y* | U |

\* women only

L = latent porphyria
NT = not tested or not published
S = symptomatic porphyria
U = uncertain (non-significant trend)
Y = yes

groups. All three retrospective studies show a global increase in renal failure in porphyric subjects. Only the Chester data are sub-divided according to porphyria activity, showing that four deaths due to renal failure were in subjects with symptomatic porphyria (the porphyria status is unknown in the fifth) (Table 3).

The Finnish study showed that low urinary PBG excretion predicts a low risk of developing symptomatic porphyria. In the Swedish study, there was a fivefold increase in PBG excretion in symptomatic compared with latent porphyria subjects, such that the authors speculated that porphyrin metabolites may be the cause of hypertension in the symptomatic group. Our Chester study (Tables 1 and 2) showed higher blood pressure and serum creatinine and lower creatinine clearance in subjects with increased haem precursor excretion, but the difference failed to reach statistical significance. Nevertheless, the suspicion remains that porphyria activity increases the risk both of hypertension and of renal impairment – but it seems certain that latent porphyrics are also at risk.

It remains uncertain whether porphyric crises, hypertension and renal damage are all independent manifestations in the severe porphyric patient by unknown or co-inherited mechanisms or whether hypertension and renal failure are causally related to porphyric 'crises' which may, however, be biochemical rather than symptomatic in some subjects (latent porphyria sufferers).

### Which is primary: hypertension or renal damage?

Although the retrospective Swedish study showed three subjects had died of chronic renal failure, the prospective study showed that no hypertensive subjects had hypertensive renal lesions. The authors speculate that this could be due either to earlier instigation of anti-hypertensive treatment or to the availability of better antihypertensive drugs than in the two Scottish studies. This conjecture implies that hypertension precedes, and subsequently causes, renal damage. Several subjects in Chester, Sweden and Finland have hypertension and normal renal function, but we believe that caution is needed in ascribing the renal damage to hypertension. The primary event could be a humoral or neurogenic insult to arterioles causing spasm; this would explain some of the manifestations of a porphyric crisis such as amblyopia, exudative or haemorrhagic retinopathy and papilloedema (Chapter 7), renal impairment and hypertension. Hypertension is not the prerequisite of any of the above, and we list some examples:

*1.5.5* (Chapter 6): latent porphyria. Died with papilloedema, meningism and coma, but was normotensive throughout. Post-mortem failed to show any intracranial pathology.

*1.9.2* (Part 4 and Chapter 7): symptomatic porphyria. Presented with scattered retinal haemorrhages when he was normotensive. He had mild renal impairment and only later became hypertensive.

*1.1.1.1* and *1.1.1.2*: siblings, both symptomatic. They were normotensive but had mild renal impairment in 1985. 1.1.1.1 has since become hypertensive (Table 3).

*1.6.5.3* (our index case): symptomatic porphyria. She had 14 severe attacks of porphyria before 1985 and occasional attacks until 1990 (Chapter 7). The crises were accompanied by transient hypertension, renal failure and hyponatraemia (Chapter 9). In between attacks she has remained normotensive, but in 1995 she had mild renal impairment for the first time (blood urea 8.7 mmol/l, creatinine 132 µmol/l). Her blood pressure is 130/85 mmHg.

*Swedish patient 1*[5]: normotensive until a severe attack of porphyria caused quadriplegia, permanent renal insufficiency and 'secondary hypertension'. Temporary bilateral visual impairment and a permanent right-sided deafness.

*Swedish patient 4*: reduced creatinine clearance, but blood pressure has never been elevated despite previous severe porphyric attacks.

*1-year old girl* (described by Whitelaw[25]): developed renal failure during an attack of porphyria. The renal impairment then persisted, although blood pressure remained normal.

The possible humoral or neurogenic insults to the kidneys and vascular system as a whole have been discussed earlier in this chapter and by others,[5,9] but Denny-Brown and Sciarra's suggestion more than 50 years ago of a locally active vasoconstrictor substance[26] has yet to be identified. Hopefully, the recent creation by Meyer's group[27] (see Chapter 7) of a genetically engineered mouse with PBG deaminase deficiency which recapitulates the drug-induced biochemical abnormalities of acute hepatic porphyria will further the cause, perhaps by testing the suggestion by Kupferschmidt *et al*[28] that decreased nitric oxide production is responsible. Literature reviews of the prevalence of hypertension and renal failure in porphyria suggest that the commonest scenario is a patient with recurrent porphyric crises complicated by transient, then sustained, hypertension and subsequent renal failure. However, the present study and review make it plain that this is not always the case, that subjects with latent porphyria are also at risk and that renal failure may precede hypertension.

## Hypertension, renal impairment and gender

Guidance on whether porphyria activity predisposes to hypertension and renal failure might be expected from a study of the gender of the persons at risk because most authors, including those in Finland,[4] have found that symptomatic porphyria is commoner in women than in men. Moore *et al*[29] summarised this view by stating that:

> *all major series show a female preponderance of symptomatic though not latent disease.*

This female preponderance is not found either in Chester (Table 3; Table 2, Chapter 7) or in Andersson and Lithner's Swedish study.[5] The Chester study found that 14 of 16 porphyric males (87%) in generation III and four of eight porphyric females (50%) were symptomatic, with approximately half of both genders having hypertension or renal failure (Tables 3 and 5). In the Swedish study half the 50 porphyric subjects had symptomatic porphyria: 17 men (8 hypertensive) and eight women (6 hypertensive) (Table 5). It was in the women that creatinine levels were higher than in matched controls. In the Finnish study,[4] all five people with porphyria who died of chronic renal failure were women; in the prospective study, the prevalence of chronic renal failure was higher than expected in women aged 30–54 years compared with age-matched women in the general Finnish population.

**Table 5.** Prevalence of hypertension and/or renal failure in 38 Chester grandchildren and 50 Swedish people according to gender and porphyria activity.

| | Chester | | | | | | | | Sweden | | | | |
| | Sympto-matic | | Latent | | Porphyria-negative | | Unknown | | Sympto-matic | | Latent | | Ratio HT/RF: |
| | No. | HT/RF | No. | HT/RF | No. | HT/RF | No. | HT/RF | No. | HT/RF | No. | HT/RF | Total |
|---|---|---|---|---|---|---|---|---|---|---|---|---|---|
| Male | 14 | 8 | 2 | 1 | 3 | 0 | 2 | 0 | 17 | 8 | 16 | 2 | 19:49 |
| Female | 4 | 2 | 4 | 2 | 6 | 0 | 3 | 0 | 8 | 6 | 9 | 2 | 12:25 |
| Total | 18 | 10 | 6 | 3 | 9 | 0 | 5 | 0 | 25 | 14 | 25 | 4 | 31:74 |

HT = hypertension
RF = renal failure

In summary, the Scandinavian surveys, but not that in Chester, suggest that hypertension and renal failure are more common in women than in men. The Finnish study, but not that in Sweden or Chester, shows symptomatic porphyria to be commoner in women. We conclude that there may be a preponderance of women developing these complications of porphyria, but in Chester the male sex has also suffered sorely. Of course, other factors may be active, including:

- the unusual biochemistry of the Chester porphyria, which perhaps worsens the male risk;
- possible demographic factors skewing the figures – the Swedish authors report a higher migration rate in women than in men, but this is not true in Chester where very few have left the city; or
- the reported differences between sexes and between series could be due to chance.

If the hypertension and renal failure are due to humoral or neurogenic effects on the vascular bed and on the kidneys, and if the sequelae are commoner in women, it is tempting to draw a pathogenetic analogy with toxaemia of pregnancy. This, however, seems improbable because subjects in the Scottish, Chester and Swedish studies with porphyria-associated renal impairment show little or no proteinuria.

Although blood pressure and renal function measurements are more complete in generation III Chester subjects than in generation IV, and notwithstanding the age difference, we believe that members of the former are more severely afflicted than their children (54% vs 28% of porphyric subjects with hypertension or renal failure; 8 deaths vs none). We attribute this to the:

- earlier discovery of hypertension in generation IV (largely as a result of our surveys);
- better and more widespread use of hypotensive medication, and
- lower prevalence of acute porphyric crises in the junior generation, doubtless helped by the demise of the barbiturate era.

## Part 4: Hypertension and chronic renal failure: case histories of afflicted members of generation III

*1.1.1*: latent porphyria. Died age 63 years of cerebellar haemorrhage and hypertension.

*1.1.5*: symptomatic porphyria. Died age 40 years in 1969 of uraemia, hypertension and acute intermittent porphyria. Six years previously his blood pressure had been 180/130 mmHg and his blood urea 110 mg% (18 mmol/l) (Chapter 5).

*1.1.6*: latent porphyria. A housewife, born in 1932, was hypertensive in both pregnancies in the mid-1950s. She presented in 1967 with cough, and a chest radiograph showed infiltration in both upper lobes suggestive of tuberculosis. Scalene node biopsy was typical of sarcoidosis. Her blood pressure was 180/110 mmHg, blood urea raised at 108–124 mg% (18–21 mmol/l), and serum calcium was raised at 10.6–12.2 mg% (2.65–3.05 mmol/l) (normal 8.5–10.5 mg%). Her urine contained protein (20 mg%) but there were no casts. She gave the history of porphyria in her brother, 1.1.5, Bekerus' index case (Chapter 5), so her urine was tested and found to contain PBG. Intravenous urogram showed both kidneys to be small. She gave no history suggestive of pyelonephritis. She was referred to Dr HJ Goldsmith, consultant nephrologist at the Liverpool Royal Infirmary, who performed renal biopsy. This showed extensive loss of renal tissue, with more than half the glomeruli replaced by compressed fibrous knots. It was uncertain whether the changes represented previous glomerulonephritis or advanced vascular nephrosclerosis. There was no evidence of renal sarcoidosis, and Goldsmith felt that the kidney in sarcoidosis would be large rather than small.

Steroid treatment was started in view of a worsening chest radiograph and persisting hypercalcaemia, and there was modest improvement in renal function. Reserpine was started in 1970 because of persisting hypertension, and later replaced by methyldopa and a thiazide diuretic. Her blood pressure remained under good control, and in 1975 her blood urea was 164 mg% (27 mmol/l), creatinine 2.4 mg% (212 µmol/l), and

24-hour urine calcium excretion 225 mg (5.6 mmol). Her serum calcium remained intermittently raised despite oral prednisolone. She was changed to propranolol, and also started on allopurinol because of persisting hyperuricaemia.

Over the last 20 years she has remained remarkably well, with no major illness. Her blood pressure has been under good control, and her serum calcium normal for some years. Her renal function has progressively deteriorated, and she started renal dialysis in 1997.

It seems certain that this patient has sarcoidosis and that the consequent hypercalcaemia has played a role in her renal failure. However, it must be remembered that she had small shrunken kidneys with nephrosclerosis from the outset. Our hypothesis is that porphyric kidney damage was the initial event, later exacerbated by hypercalcaemia due to coincidental sarcoidosis. The patient had hyperuricaemia, assumed secondary to the renal failure. She has not experienced clinical gout or nephrolithiasis, her urine has never contained granular casts and was usually negative for protein. No other member of the kindred has been noted to have sarcoidosis or hypercalcaemia.

*1.2.1*: died age 29 years in 1946 of uraemia and nephritis.

*1.2.8*: his brother, died age 18 years in 1953 of left ventricular failure and malignant hypertension.

*1.2*: their father, died age 62 years in 1953 of obstructive airways disease and hypertension.

It is not known whether any of these members had symptomatic porphyria (Chapter 6).

*1.6.3* (her story is recorded in Chapter 4): died age 46 years in 1978 at the Chester City Hospital. She presented in 1954 at the age of 23 years with an acute porphyric crisis, hypertension (180/110 mmHg), papilloedema and renal failure with blood urea 111 mg% (18 mmol/l). She remained hypertensive, and treatment with guanethidine was started in 1967 when her blood urea was 44–105 mg% (7–17 mmol/l) and her average urea clearance 21% of normal. Urine testing was negative for protein. She remained on guanethidine until her final admission with a dense stroke from which she died before blood tests for renal function could be performed. Necropsy showed cerebellar haemorrhage, enlargement of the left cardiac ventricle and small shrunken kidneys with granular subcapsular surfaces. Histology showed considerable loss of renal cortex with sclerosed and acellular glomeruli. The arterioles showed marked thickening of the walls and luminal narrowing, with marked fibrinoid necrosis indicative of renal hypertensive damage. Renal histology at necropsy was similar to that of the renal biopsy in her cousin, 1.1.6.

Her mother, 1.6, who had positive urine and faecal tests for porphyria, lived to 81 despite hypertension reported to Bekerus and recorded in the family history section of her daughter's hospital case-notes. Her daughter, 1.6.3.2, who is porphyria-positive, has a blood pressure of 120/70 mmHg (1995 measurement).

*1.6.5*: symptomatic porphyria. Died of cerebral haemorrhage, malignant hypertension and porphyria at the age of 37. He had hypertension and uraemia at the age of 19 years during a porphyric crisis (Chapter 6).

*1.8.3*: died age 47 years in 1982 at the Chester City Hospital. She had 12 children in two marriages and was hypertensive during her pregnancies from at least 1965 when 'the puerperium was complicated by raised blood pressure somewhat alleviated by sedation'. In 1969 and 1970 she was taking phenobarbitone 30 mg tds and Navidrex K (cyclopenthiazide and potassium chloride). She was referred by the consultant obstetrician, Mr Sol Bender, from the postnatal clinic in 1973 to Dr PI Adnitt, consultant physician, because of persisting hypertension (180/120 mmHg). Her blood urea was 56 mg% (9 mmol/l). Her urine was sterile and free of protein or casts. She defaulted from follow-up and received no treatment. She remained well until admitted in her final illness with a blood pressure of 180/110 mmHg, urea 52.6 mmol/l, and creatinine 1,368 µmol/l. Her urine was again normal on culture and microscopy. She died seven days later. Necropsy was not performed.

*1.9.2*: symptomatic porphyria. An unemployed labourer, he died age 55 years in 1988 in the Countess of Chester Hospital. He had a history of abdominal pain and red urine, and porphyria was confirmed by Bekerus in 1964. He presented in 1977 with failing vision and acute gout. Scattered retinal haemorrhages were seen (Chapter 7). His blood pressure was 140/80 mmHg. On three occasions his urine contained no protein, casts or red or white cells. His blood urea was 10 mmol/l, creatinine 137 µmol/l, and uric acid 0.62 mmol/l. A year later, without treatment, urea was normal and uric acid 0.59 mmol/l. In 1979, he developed hypertension, and was started on propranolol, 160 mg daily, and allopurinol. His retinal haemorrhages persisted, blood urea was 8.4 mmol/l, creatinine 152 µmol/l and creatinine clearance 11 ml/min. Intravenous urogram showed poor concentration by kidneys that were probably small. Blood pressure control was poor. In 1982, he had a brief porphyric crisis with abdominal pain and vomiting. Later the same year, he developed wheezing thought to be due to propranolol which was, therefore, changed to indoramin which was continued for two years. At about this time he became very restless and agitated and was started on chlorpromazine 100 mg nocte, which he took for at least a year.

In 1983, he was admitted because of tardive dyskinesia and akathisia which was a great tribulation to him and his family, but which was unresponsive to medication. His blood urea was 15.7 mmol/l and creatinine 368 µmol/l. His blood pressure control remained poor and his renal

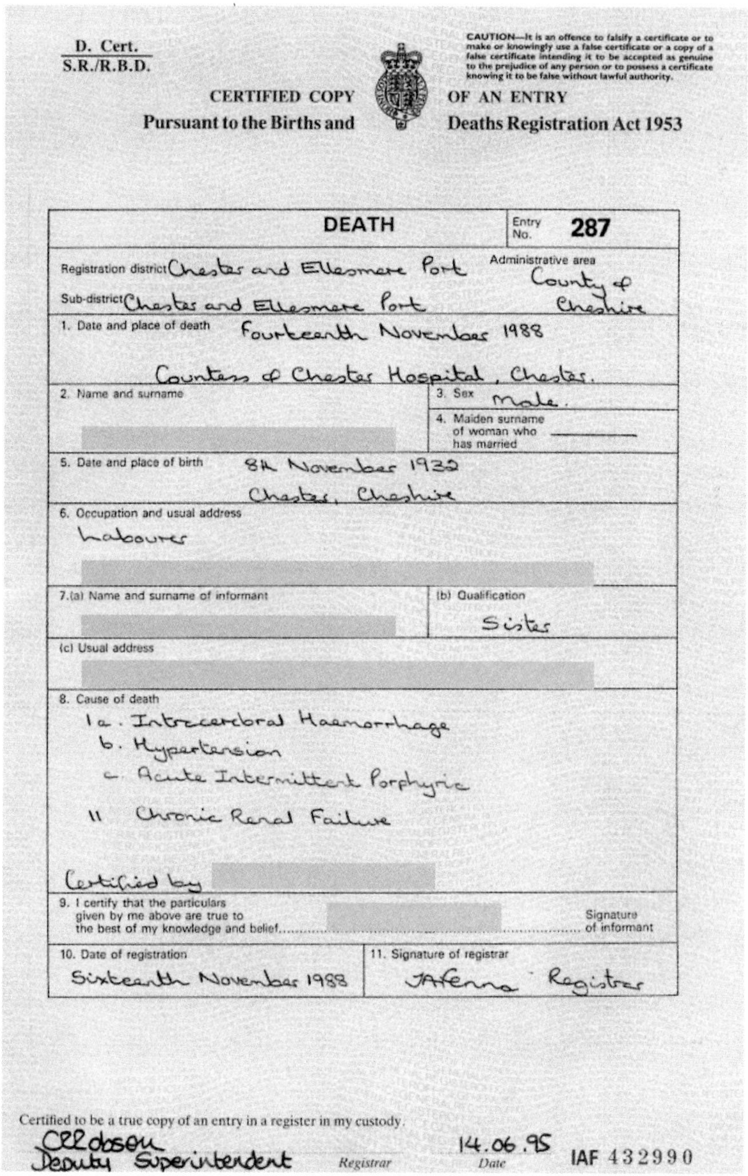

CAUTION—It is an offence to falsify a certificate or to make or knowingly use a false certificate or a copy of a false certificate intending it to be accepted as genuine to the prejudice of any person or to possess a certificate knowing it to be false without lawful authority.

D. Cert.
S.R./R.B.D.

CERTIFIED COPY OF AN ENTRY
Pursuant to the Births and Deaths Registration Act 1953

**DEATH**    Entry No. **287**

Registration district Chester and Ellesmere Port    Administrative area County of

Sub-district Chester and Ellesmere Port    Cheshire

1. Date and place of death   Fourteenth November 1988

Countess of Chester Hospital, Chester.

2. Name and surname    3. Sex Male.

4. Maiden surname of woman who has married

5. Date and place of birth   8th November 1932

Chester, Cheshire

6. Occupation and usual address   Labourer

7.(a) Name and surname of informant    (b) Qualification Sister

(c) Usual address

8. Cause of death

   1 a. Intracerebral Haemorrhage

   b. Hypertension

   c. Acute Intermittent Porphyria

   II   Chronic Renal Failure

Certified by

9. I certify that the particulars given by me above are true to the best of my knowledge and belief..........    Signature of informant

10. Date of registration   Sixteenth November 1988    11. Signature of registrar   JAFenna Registrar

Certified to be a true copy of an entry in a register in my custody.

CRobson Deputy Superintendent   Registrar   14.06.95 Date   IAF 432990

**Fig 2.** Death certificate of subject 1.9.2.

function continued to deteriorate. He was referred to the regional renal unit in 1986 where an isotope scan showed a normal right kidney but a very small left kidney. Dr JM Bone, consultant nephrologist, opined:

*If he had more in the way of degenerative vascular disease, I would be tempted to suggest that his small left kidney had originated from such a cause and was secondary to his hypertension. He may, however, have had a small kidney all along. The combination of uric acid nephropathy and hypertensive nephrosclerosis is, of course, well known to us, but generally does not progress so rapidly.*

Later the same year he developed a severe motor neuropathy which required hospital admission for six months. His blood pressure control improved considerably during this stay, and may explain why his blood urea of 68.4 mmol/l improved to 21 mmol/l and his creatinine from 724 µmol/l to 464 µmol/l. We speculated that aluminium hydroxide, listed as being unsafe in porphyria,[30] prescribed as a phosphate binder may have precipitated the severe porphyric neuropathy. This was therefore replaced by calcium carbonate, but on two occasions it was followed by intense pruritus. In 1988, he was started on haemodialysis pending a renal transplant, and over the next few months developed bullous lesions on his fingertips (Fig 1, Chapter 7), gynaecomastia, vitreous haemorrhage and extension of his central and peripheral retinal haemorrhages, and recurrent ascites. He was finally admitted later that year with an extensive cerebrovascular accident. Death was certified as due to intracerebral haemorrhage, hypertension, acute intermittent porphyria and chronic renal failure (Fig 2).

As in other members of the family with impaired renal function, it is difficult to know whether hypertension or renal disease was the primary event. We suspect the latter, as on presentation the patient was normotensive but had renal impairment. Similarly, it is difficult to say whether the hyperuricaemia was primary or secondary and, if primary, what role it played in the progressive renal disease. There was no evidence of complication by renal calculi. In retrospect, it is possible that the restlessness and agitation he developed in 1981 was an extrapyramidal side effect of the indoramin – a known hazard,[30] although we have found no case reports in the literature to substantiate this. Ridley[31] points out that restlessness and insomnia can presage a porphyric attack. It is sad and ironic that chlorpromazine, well-known for its extrapyramidal side effects, was chosen to treat the agitation and probably exacerbated the akathisia.[32]

# References

1 Qadiri MR, Church SE, McColl KEL, Moore MR, Youngs GR. Chester porphyria: a clinical study of a new form of acute porphyria. *British Medical Journal* 1986; **292**: 455–9.
2 Church SE. *The Chester porphyria*. MD Thesis, University of Liverpool, 1986.
3 Church SE, McColl KE, Moore MR, Youngs GR. Hypertension and renal impairment as complications of acute porphyria. *Nephrology Dialysis Transplantation* 1992; **7**: 986–90.
4 Kauppinen R, Mustajoki P. Prognosis of acute porphyria: occurrence of acute attacks, precipitating factors, and associated diseases. *Medicine* 1992; **71**: 1–13.

5  Andersson C, Lithner F. Hypertension and renal disease in patients with acute intermittent porphyria. *Journal of Internal Medicine* 1994; **236**: 169–75.

6  Goldberg A. Acute intermittent porphyria: a study of 50 cases. *Quarterly Journal of Medicine* 1959; NS **28**: 183–209.

7  Eales L, Day RS, Blekkenhorst GH. The clinical and biochemical features of variegate porphyria: an analysis of 300 cases studied at Groote Schuur Hospital, Cape Town. *International Journal of Biochemistry* 1980; **12**: 837–53.

8  Beattie AD, Goldberg A. Acute intermittent porphyria: natural history and prognosis. In: Doss M (ed). *Porphyrins in human diseases*. Basel: Karger, 1976: 245–50.

9  Yeung Laiwah ACC, Mactier R, McColl KEL, Moore MR, Goldberg A. Early onset chronic renal failure as a complication of acute intermittent porphyria. *Quarterly Journal of Medicine* 1983; **205**: 92–8.

10  McColl KEL, Thompson GG, Moore MR, Goldberg A, *et al*. Chester porphyria: biochemical studies of a new form of acute porphyria. *Lancet* 1985; ii: 796–9.

11  O'Brien E, Mee F, Atkins N, O'Malley K. Inaccuracy of the Hawksley random zero sphygmomanometer. *Lancet* 1990; **336**: 1465–8.

12  Alderman MH. The epidemiology of hypertension: etiology, natural history, and the impact of therapy. *Cardiovascular Reviews and Reports* 1980; **1**: 509–19.

13  Kezdi P. Neurogenic hypertension in man in porphyria. *American Medical Association Archives of Internal Medicine* 1954; **94**: 122–30.

14  Oakley CM (editorial). The heart in the Guillain-Barré syndrome. *British Medical Journal* 1984; **288**: 94.

15  McDowell FH, Plum F. Arterial hypertension associated with acute anterior poliomyelitis. *New England Journal of Medicine* 1951; **245**: 241–5.

16  Gibson JB, Goldberg A. The neuropathology of acute porphyria. *Journal of Pathology and Bacteriology* 1956; **71**: 495–509.

17  Talman WT, Snyder D, Reis DJ. Chronic lability of arterial pressure produced by destruction of A2 catecholaminergic neurons in rat brainstem. *Circulation Research* 1980; **46**: 842–53.

18  Mustajoki P, Seppäläinen AM. Neuropathy in latent hereditary hepatic porphyria. *British Medical Journal* 1975; **2**: 310–2.

19  Heilmann E, Muller KN. Clinical and morphological aspects of acute intermittent porphyria. In: Doss M (ed). *Porphyrins in human diseases*. Basel: Karger, 1976: 282–5.

20  Campbell JAH. The pathology of the South African genetic porphyria. *South African Journal of Laboratory and Clinical Medicine* 1963; **9**: 197–203.

21  Ivanov E, Todorov D, Adjarov D, Dimitrov P. Porphyrin metabolism in renal diseases. *Nephron* 1976; **17**: 396–401.

22  Day RS, Eales L, Disler PB. Porphyrias and the kidney (editorial). *Nephron* 1981; **28**: 261–7.

23 Campbell BC, Beattie AD, Moore MR, Goldberg A, Reid AG. Renal insufficiency associated with excessive lead exposure. *British Medical Journal* 1977; **1**: 482–5.

24 McColl KEL, Moore MR, Thompson GG, Goldberg A. Screening for latent acute intermittent porphyria: the value of measuring both leucocyte δ-aminolaevulinic acid synthase and erythrocyte uroporphyrinogen-1-synthase activities. *Journal of Medical Genetics* 1982; **19**: 271–6.

25 Whitelaw AGL. Acute intermittent porphyria, hypercholesterolaemia and renal impairment. *Archives of Disease in Childhood* 1974; **49**: 406–7.

26 Denny-Brown D, Sciarra D. Changes in the nervous system in acute porphyria. *Brain* 1945; **68**: 1–16.

27 Lindberg RLP, Porcher G, Grandchamp B, Ledermann B, *et al*. Porphobilinogen deaminase deficiency in mice causes a neuropathy resembling that of human hepatic porphyria (letter). *Nature Genetics* 1996; **12**: 195–9.

28 Kupferschmidt H, Bont A, Schnorf H, Landis T, *et al*. Transient cortical blindness and bioccipital brain lesions in two patients with acute intermittent porphyria. *Annals of Internal Medicine* 1995; **123**: 598–600.

29 Moore MR, McColl KEL, Rimington C, Goldberg A. *Disorders of porphyrin metabolism*. New York: Plenum, 1987.

30 *British National Formulary*. London: British Medical Association and Royal Pharmaceutical Society, 1995.

31 Ridley A. The neuropathy of acute intermittent porphyria. *Quarterly Journal of Medicine* 1969; **38** NS: 307–33.

32 Anonymous. Akathisia and antipsychotic drugs. *Lancet* 1986; **ii**: 1131–2.

*Chapter 9*

# Hyponatraemia frequently complicates acute porphyric crises

DAVID CHEW, SUSAN CHURCH AND
GILES YOUNGS

Hyponatraemia has been recognised as a complication of acute porphyric crisis,[1-3] but its incidence and severity are probably greater than is realised by the physician with only occasional contact with the disease. Although the cause of the hyponatraemia is controversial, iatrogenic factors may be contributory, especially intravenous fluid therapy. We have studied retrospectively the occurrence of hyponatraemia in 31 acute porphyric crises in two members of the Chester kindred (1.6.5.3, 1.8.3.3), and related this to the volumes of intravenous fluids infused.

## Subjects and methods

The case-notes and records of fluid balance were studied for two female patients admitted with 31 separate episodes of porphyric crisis over an eight-year period (1977–85). Both subjects belonged to generation IV of the Chester kindred:

*1.8.3.3*: admitted on 17 occasions between 1977 and 1981, when she died aged 25 years of respiratory paralysis during an acute crisis.

*1.6.5.3*: admitted on 14 occasions between 1981 (age 15 years) and 1985; she is now 30 years old and remains well.

The acute attacks followed a common pattern, with ill-defined pain in the limbs, loins and abdomen, profound misery, constipation and occasional vomiting. Neither medication nor alcohol has been implicated as a precipitant, but attacks often began premenstrually (Chapters 6 and 7). Hyponatraemia was defined as a serum sodium less than 135 mmol/l (moderate: 125-134 mmol/l; severe: <125 mmol/l).

## Results

Serum sodium was measured on arrival at hospital on 26 of the 31 admissions for acute porphyric crisis; it was normal on 21 occasions (81%) and moderately low on the others. During the period of each admission the serum sodium remained normal in only 12 of the 27 occasions (44%) when it was measured. Hyponatraemia complicated the remaining 15 admissions (56%), with severe hyponatraemia (serum sodium <125 mmol/l) during eight. The initial sodium was normal on five of these eight occasions, there was moderate hyponatraemia in two, and it was not measured in the other. The time taken for the serum sodium to reach its nadir was 2–10 days (average: 4 days), but neither the rate of fall nor the maximum degree of hyponatraemia seemed related to the serum sodium on admission.

Records of fluids infused intravenously were available for only five of the eight admissions complicated by severe hyponatraemia. During four of these, all in the early part of the study period, there was modest overinfusion of intravenous fluids (average: 3.4 litres over the 24 hours prior to the lowest level of serum sodium). Both patients experienced convulsions on one occasion, the serum sodium being 115 mmol/l and 114 mmol/l, respectively. In the latter part of the study period, they were both treated with fluid restriction, despite vomiting, oliguria and rising blood urea.

An example of the changes observed in serum sodium and urea levels during one admission in the latter part of the study is shown in Fig 1. Fluid intake was restricted to an average of 1.5 l/24 hours but, despite this, serum sodium fell to 121 mmol/l and 120 mmol/l by the 10th and 15th days, respectively. Urinary sodium levels during the period of most severe hyponatraemia averaged 32 mmol/l daily. Urine osmolality was always substantially higher than serum osmolality at this time, and the osmolality gap (the difference between actual and calculated serum osmolality), measured on three occasions, was less than 10 mOsmol/kg. More rigorous fluid restriction to only 500 ml/24 hours was instituted on days 16–21 despite the rising blood urea and oliguria. Serum sodium then rose rapidly *pari passu* with clinical improvement and reduced opiate requirements.

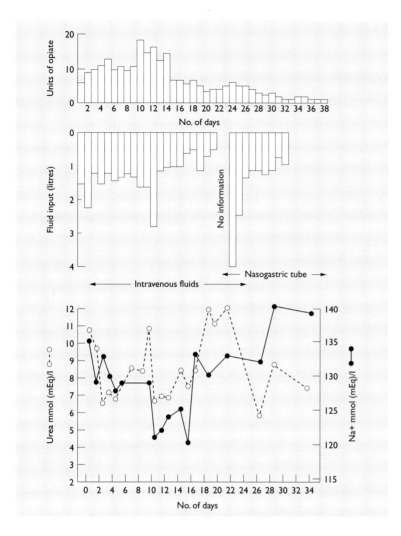

Fig 1. Subject 1.6.5.3: serum sodium and fluid intake during hospital admission with acute porphyric crisis (units of opiate indicate severity of symptoms; 1 unit = 15 mg morphine rectally or 50 mg pethidine intramuscularly).

## Discussion

Our study demonstrates that hyponatraemia is a common complication of the acute porphyric crisis. Eales *et al*[3] in a study of 45 acute attacks of variegate porphyria found hyponatraemia in 58% of attacks on admission and in a further 37% after admission, with an elevated blood urea at some time in 91% of the attacks.

The cause of the electrolyte disturbance remains controversial, and several factors may be involved. Among the suggested mechanisms are:

- extrarenal loss by vomiting or diarrhoea,[2,3]
- failure of the kidney to excrete a water load because of inappropriate secretion of antidiuretic hormone (ADH),[2,4] or
- an intrinsic tubular defect.[3,5]

139

Other possibilities include the so-called sick-cell syndrome and a resetting of the osmoreceptor response[6] as occurs in the Guillain-Barré syndrome which, like porphyria, can be complicated by hyponatraemia, transient hypertension and tachycardia.

In our subjects, vomiting was not severe and diarrhoea was never seen, making extrarenal sodium loss an unlikely explanation for the hyponatraemia, especially as daily urine sodium concentration in the example shown in Fig 1 averaged 32 mmol/l. It also seems unlikely that sick-cell syndrome caused the hyponatraemia as the associated osmolality gap which usually occurs in that situation[7] was absent on the three occasions it was measured in our study. Neither subject experienced excess thirst – rather the opposite, in that they often refused to drink.

The patients tended to secrete a relatively concentrated urine, which would suggest a defect in water excretion, which could either be renal in origin or secondary to increased production of ADH. The latter may represent either a specific abnormality of ADH metabolism or a rather non-specific response in severely ill patients given opiates.[8] However, blood urea was elevated in our two subjects, which would be unusual in a pure case of inappropriate secretion of ADH in which urea is usually very low as a result of dilution.[3] ADH levels were not measured in our subjects, but levels of the hormone were shown by Zerbe et al[9] during the study period (1977–85) to correlate poorly with the hyponatraemia. They found normal plasma ADH levels in 80% of a group of 79 patients with apparent inappropriate ADH secretion. The interpretation of the role of ADH is further complicated by the observation that some patients have abnormally low blood volumes,[10] so that any increased release of the hormone is appropriate rather than inappropriate, and is mediated by volume receptors. The combination of a low sodium and a high urea suggests impairment of the kidney's capacity to excrete a water load, perhaps as a result of some form of acute toxic effect on the diluting segment.[3] It has now been recognised that acute porphyria can be complicated by chronic renal failure and hypertension (Chapter 8),[11,12] indicating that renal involvement is part of the porphyric syndrome.

In the early part of the study period, the dangers of infusing even modest quantities of fluids for rehydration, as advocated by Waldenström,[13] were underappreciated. Overinfusion of fluid was clearly a contributory factor causing hyponatraemia. However, it also occurred later despite moderate fluid restriction, and was only corrected by rigorous restriction of fluids. This may suggest both a renal tubular defect and inappropriate secretion of ADH.

The porphyric subject is at risk of being given a fluid load, both because there are clinical signs of dehydration, and also because standard advice is that a high carbohydrate intake is beneficial by blocking the induction of delta-aminolaevulinic acid synthase, the rate-limiting enzyme in the haem biosynthetic pathway.[14] Our patients' refusal to drink, poor venous access and the impracticality of repeated insertion of central venous catheters because of the frequency of admission, make it difficult to follow the standard advice of glucose drinks or 20% laevulose infusions through a central line.[14,15] Whenever possible, a fine-bore nasogastric tube is passed, but it has been necessary to fashion an arteriovenous fistula in one of the two subjects.

Acute porphyria is a rare disease, and most physicians will rarely, if ever, see a case of acute porphyric crisis. The life-threatening complication of motor neuropathy leading to respiratory or bulbar palsy is well recognised, but hyponatraemia is a more common complication with a considerable morbidity, particularly convulsions probably due to cerebral oedema.[16,17] Although the cause of the electrolyte disturbance is poorly understood, it is undoubtedly exacerbated by even moderate fluid administration and helped by fluid restriction. The optimum treatment of hyponatraemia remains controversial; some people advocate rapid correction,[18] while others advocate a more conservative approach, feeling that rapid correction leads to central pontine myelinolysis.[19]

We feel that these therapeutic implications for porphyria have been insufficiently emphasised hitherto. Meticulous attention should be given to fluid balance, and strict fluid restriction instituted in the event of hyponatraemia even in the presence of oliguria and a rising blood urea.

## References

1 Linder GC. Salt metabolism in acute porphyria. Report of two cases. *Lancet* 1947; **ii**: 649–52.

2 Ludwig GD, Goldberg M. Hyponatremia in acute intermittent porphyria probably resulting from inappropriate secretion of antidiuretic hormone. *Annals of the New York Academy of Sciences* 1963; **104**: 710–34.

3 Eales L, Dowdle EB, Sweeney GD. The acute porphyric attack. I. The electrolyte disorder of the acute porphyric attack and the possible role of delta-aminolaevulinic acid. *South African Journal of Laboratory and Clinical Medicine* (special issue) 1971; 25 September:89-97.

4 Hellman ES, Tschudy DP, Bartter FC. Abnormal electrolyte and water metabolism in acute intermittent porphyria. The transient inappropriate secretion of antidiuretic hormone. *American Journal of Medicine* 1962; **32**: 734–46.

5 Eales L, Day RS, Blekkenhorst GH. The clinical and biochemical features of variegate porphyria: an analysis of 300 cases studied at Groote Schuur Hospital, Cape Town. *International Journal of Biochemistry* 1980; **12**: 837–53.

6 Penney MD, Murphy D, Walters G. Resetting of osmoreceptor response as cause of hyponatraemia in acute idiopathic polyneuritis. *British Medical Journal* 1979; **2**: 1474–6.

7 Flear CTG, Gill GV. Hyponatraemia: mechanisms and management. Lancet 1981; **ii**: 26–31.

8 Fujimoto JM. The kidney: sites of action of narcotic analgesic drugs. In: Clouet DH (ed). *Narcotic drugs: biochemical pharmacology.* New York: Plenum, 1971: 366–7.

9 Zerbe R, Stropes L, Robertson G. Vasopressin function in the syndrome of inappropriate antidiuresis. *Annual Review of Medicine* 1980; **31**: 315–27.

10 Bloomer JR, Berk PD, Bonkowsky HL, Stein JA, *et al.* Blood volume and bilirubin production in acute intermittent porphyria. *New England Journal of Medicine* 1971; **284**: 17–20.

11 Yeung Liawah AAC, Mactier R, McColl KEL, Moore MR, Goldberg A. Early onset chronic renal failure as a complication of acute intermittent porphyria. *Quarterly Journal of Medicine* 1983; **205**: 92–8.

12 Church SE, McColl KE, Moore MR, Youngs GR. Hypertension and renal impairment as complications of acute porphyria. *Nephrology Dialysis Transplantation* 1992; **7**: 986–90.

13 Waldenström J. The porphyrias as inborn errors of metabolism. *American Journal of Medicine* 1957; **22**: 758–73.

14 Brodie MJ, Moore MR, Thompson GG, Goldberg A. The treatment of acute intermittent porphyria with laevulose. *Clinical Science and Molecular Medicine* 1977; **53**: 365–71.

15 Moore MR, McColl KEL, Rimington C, Goldberg A. *Disorders of porphyria metabolism.* New York: Plenum, 1987.

16 Arieff AI. Hyponatraemia, convulsions, respiratory arrest, and permanent brain damage after elective surgery in healthy women. *New England Journal of Medicine* 1986; **314**: 1529–35.

17 Ellis SJ. Severe hyponatraemia: complications and treatment. *Quarterly Journal of Medicine* 1995; **88**: 905–9.

18 Arieff AI. Management of hyponatraemia. *British Medical Journal* 1993; **307**: 305–8.

19 Sterns RH. The treatment of hyponatraemia: first, do no harm. *American Journal of Medicine* 1990: **88**; 557–60.

*Chapter 10*

# Asthma and atopy in the kindred: a surrogate marker for Chester porphyria?

TUDOR TOMA, JONATHAN EVANS, JOANNA SAYER
AND GILES YOUNGS

It was shown in Chapter 8 that chronic hypertension and renal failure occur only in the porphyric members of the Chester kindred, and that their presence might therefore act as a marker for porphyria. Thus, in deceased subjects whose medical records have been destroyed, knowledge of hypertension and renal failure from a death certificate, like knowledge of paralysis, provides circumstantial evidence of porphyria. In only four subjects, the brothers 1.2.1, 1.2.3, 1.2.4 and 1.2.8 (Chapter 6), has such circumstantial evidence been used to assign porphyric status, but in the same chapter we suggest that such evidence supports the hypothesis that all Peter Dobson's 10 children had porphyria.

In her MD thesis,[1] Church noted a high prevalence of asthma in the pedigree. All the asthmatic members she met also had porphyria. She speculated that the two conditions might be co-inherited, just as Meissner[2] had referred to co-inheritance of other dominantly inherited disorders in variegate porphyria in South Africa.

Together with eczema and hay fever, the inherited form of asthma is one of the manifestations of atopy. It is labelled 'extrinsic' asthma because atopic people are allergic to substances in the environment such as pollen or house-dust mite. Cookson *et al* showed in 1989[3,4] that the atopy gene is dominantly inherited and lies on chromosome 11q. Asthma in older people is known as 'intrinsic' asthma; it is not precipitated by naturally occurring external allergens, is associated with nasal polyps and aspirin sensitivity, and does not appear to be inherited.

There is a high prevalence of asthma in the Chester kindred, and our interest in Church's speculation that asthma and porphyria could be co-inherited in them was heightened when Norton *et al*[5,6] showed that the gene for Chester porphyria also lies on the long arm of chromosome 11q. If the genetic loci of both atopy and Chester porphyria lie close together on chromosome 11q, this could explain any coincidence of the two conditions in our family. Atopy is an easy condition to diagnose by skin-prick testing at any age, whereas children cannot be tested for porphyria because their porphobilinogen deaminase levels are usually normal regardless of porphyria status. If atopy is a marker for Chester porphyria, atopy testing could be a useful surrogate test for Chester porphyria, especially in children. A decision was taken in 1995 to test the hypothesis that atopy and Chester porphyria are co-inherited.

## Subjects and methods

A letter was sent to the 154 adult members of the Chester porphyria kindred, nearly all of whom still live in or near Chester, explaining the frequent occurrence of asthma in the family, and inviting them to attend, together with their children over the age of seven years, for tests of atopy and lung function. Failure to reply was followed 4–6 weeks later by a telephone call. Subjects were divided into two groups:

- those attending for the clinical study, and
- those who did not attend, but whose history was subsequently reviewed for evidence of asthma and atopy.

### Clinical study

The 65 subjects (52%) who attended were invited to fill out a questionnaire which included questions about smoking and medication history, and family history of asthma or wheeze. The opportunity was taken to update our porphyria register by recording recent marriages, births and deaths. The measurements performed are listed below. In most cases, the investigator was unaware of the porphyria status of the subject:

- *Body weight and height.*
- *Blood pressure*: recorded at the beginning and end of the attendance (using the method described in Chapter 8).
- *Spirometry*: forced expiratory volume at one second (FEV$_1$), and peak flow rate before and 15 min after an inhalation of two puffs (200 µg) of salbutamol via a spacer.
- *Skin-prick* testing was performed to house dust, house-dust mite

(*Dermatophagoides pteronyssinus*), mixed grass pollen, cat and dog dander, feathers, with a positive and negative control using a standard procedure.[7] Weal diameters were calculated minus the negative control. A test was considered positive to an allergen if the diameter was equal to or greater than that of the positive control. The test result was considered negative if the response to the negative control was greater than to the positive control or if an allergen produced a diameter equal to that of the negative control.

- *Blood* was taken to estimate haemoglobin, white cell count, automated eosinophil count, urea, creatinine, immunoglobulin (Ig) E and porphobilinogen deaminase.
- *Atopy positivity*: two or more of the following criteria were required:
  - history of asthma (intermittent wheeze starting below the age of 20 years which needed treatment) or hay fever needing treatment (in the non-clinical study, a subject was deemed to be atopic if either of these were present);
  - more than 15% reversibility with salbutamol on respiratory function tests;
  - one or more positive skin-prick tests;
  - IgE greater than two standard deviations above normal.

### Non-clinical study

The hospital case-notes of the 59 subjects (48%) who did not attend were scanned for evidence of early-onset asthma or hay fever severe enough to require treatment. About half were questioned on the telephone. Information for several others was provided by relatives attending the clinical study, and some enquiries were made to general practitioners.

### Statistical analysis

Porphyria-positive and -negative subjects were compared non-parametrically by the Mann-Whitney U-test. Contingency table analysis, odds ratios and 95% confidence intervals were estimated by exact methods (Microsoft Excel 4.0).

## Results

### Clinical study

Sixty-five subjects (37 female) attended the clinical study, of whom 21 (32%) were porphyria-positive, 24 (37%) porphyria-negative, and 20 (31%) of unknown porphyria status. Most of those of

**Table 1.** Clinical study: demography and results of lung function and atopy in 45 porphyria-positive and -negative subjects.

|  | Porphyria-positive | Porphyria-negative |
|---|---|---|
| **All subjects** | | |
| No. of subjects | 21 | 24 |
| Female | 14 | 14 |
| Average age (years) | 40 | 36 |
| Cigarette smokers | 13 (62%) | 12 (50%) |
| History of asthma | 5 (24%) | 4 (17%) |
| Mean $FEV_1$ (litres) | 271 | 311 |
| Mean $FEV_1$ increase after salbutamol (litres) | 50 (19%) | 38 (12%) |
| Mean PFR (l/min) | 429 | 476 |
| Mean PFR increase after salbutamol (l/min) | 20 (5%) | 18 (4%) |
| No. of subjects showing 15% reversibility of $FEV_1$ after salbutamol | 9 (43%) | 8 (33%) |
| Positive skin tests | 12/16 (75%) | 16/24 (67%) |
| Mean IgE (ku/l) | 49 | 58 |
| **Non-smoking subjects** | | |
| No. of subjects | 8 | 12 |
| Mean $FEV_1$ (litres) | 317 | 307 |
| No. of subjects showing 15% reversibility of $FEV_1$ after salbutamol | 1 | 5 |

$FEV_1$ = forced expiratory volume at 1 sec
IgE = immunoglobulin E
PFR = peak flow rate

unknown status were children in whom porphobilinogen deaminase levels are not useful in status designation.

Demographic details, and results of tests of lung function and atopy for the 45 porphyria-positive and -negative subjects and a subset of 20 non-smoking individuals are shown in Table 1. The groups are of similar size and gender. There were more smokers in the porphyria-positive than in the porphyria-negative subjects (62% vs 50%), and the former had slightly worse lung function. A similar proportion of both groups showed a 15% increase in $FEV_1$ after inhaling salbutamol. Mean IgE levels were more than twice as high in subjects with positive skin tests (71 ku/l) than in those with negative skin tests (31 ku/l), but there was no difference in either serum IgE levels or eosinophil counts between porphyric and non-porphyric subjects. Lung function in the non-smoking

**Table 2**. Atopy status in 124 members of the Chester porphyria kindred (combined clinical and non-clinical study).

| Porphyria status | Subjects | | |
| | Total | Atopic | |
| | | No. | % |
|---|---|---|---|
| Positive | 39 | 10 | 27 |
| Negative | 57 | 13 | 23 |
| Unknown | 28 | 7 | 25 |

porphyria-positive and -negative groups was similar, although more of the latter showed 15% reversibility after inhaling salbutamol (5 vs 1). The results for the 18 subjects of unknown porphyria status are not shown separately in Table 1, but the atopy results are included in Table 2.

### Non-clinical study

Of the 59 subjects who did not attend, 18 were porphyria-positive (30%) and 33 porphyria-negative (56%). There were eight of unknown status (14%). Atopy status, judged by a history of asthma or hay fever needing treatment, was similar in all three groups.

### Combined clinical and non-clinical study

The prevalence of atopy according to porphyria status is shown in Table 2 for all 124 subjects and was similar in the three groups. There were no statistically significant differences between porphyria and non-porphyria subjects for any of the parameters shown in Tables 1 and 2. No association was found between atopy and gender, symptomatic or latent porphyria, blood pressure or renal function.

## Discussion

Our study shows no evidence that atopy and Chester porphyria are co-inherited. The prevalence of clinical asthma in 12 of the 65 subjects (18%) in the clinical study is higher than the 6% prevalence expected in the general population.[8,9] More porphyria-positive subjects smoked cigarettes than porphyria-negative subjects (62% vs 50%), which could explain their poorer lung function and increased bronchial reactivity. The response to inhaled salbutamol was similar in both groups.

All but two of the 12 asthmatics in the clinical study had positive skin tests, and their asthma is thus probably atopic and inherited (allergic or extrinsic asthma). As recorded in Chapter 6, Peter Dobson, the fisherman, progenitor of over 300 offspring to date, was asthmatic and may have passed the atopy gene to his offspring. The picture is confused, though, because six porphyric family members (1.1.5, 1.6.1, 1.6.2, 1.6.5, 1.1.1.1, 1.9.1.2) have nasal polyps, and four of them have asthma. Their asthma could therefore be intrinsic, non-allergic asthma. However, four of the six with nasal polyps who had skin tests (1.6.1, 1.6.2, 1.1.1.1, 1.9.1.2) are positive to one or more allergens, and one of the three tested has a raised IgE.

We conclude that these subjects have both nasal polyps, with a potential for intrinsic, non-allergic asthma, and atopy, with a potential for extrinsic allergic asthma. Subjects 1.6.1, 1.6.2 and 1.6.5 are siblings, but we can find no reference in the literature to intrinsic asthma or nasal polyps being inherited – except for a report of a weak association between aspirin-induced asthma and HLA-DQw2.[10] Our six family members with nasal polyps all have porphyria, but the kindred (particularly the porphyria-negative members) have not been formally screened for nasal polyps. However, none of the three daughters of 1.6.5, who was asthmatic and had a porphyric crisis after surgery for nasal polyps (Chapter 6), has nasal polyps. One daughter (1.6.5.3), our 1980 index case, has porphyria, asthma and positive skin tests.

The seemingly high prevalence of asthma and nasal polyps in the family is intriguing, as is the uncertainty in the literature about the connection between nasal polyps, allergic and non-allergic asthma. On the one hand, the incidence of allergy in nasal polyposis patients is not different from the general population[11-13] while, on the other, peripheral blood and bronchial mucosal eosinophilia is a prominent feature of both allergic and non-allergic asthma.[14,15] In nasal polyposis, with or without asthma, there is an elevation of peripheral blood eosinophil count that is independent of allergy.[16]

## Conclusion

There is insufficient evidence to link nasal polyps with Chester porphyria or to show whether they are co-inherited in the kindred. We think the kindred provides an ideal crucible for a study of the interrelationships of nasal polyps, asthma and atopy. Perhaps this is peripheral to our interest in porphyria – or maybe not, because who knows what heritable links might be shown? It is ironic that the dominantly inherited atopy is not co-inherited with porphyria, despite the genes for both lying on the same chromosome, while hypertension, which has a less well defined and probably polygenic inheritance in the general population, is closely linked with porphyria in our family. This suggests that the hypertension and renal failure in our family is a consequence of porphyria. Fascinating though these speculations may be, it is disappointing that atopy has not proven to be a surrogate marker for Chester porphyria.

*Acknowledgement*

We express our thanks to Professor George Elder, University of Wales, for testing the blood samples.

# References

1  Church SE. *The Chester porphyria*. MD Thesis, University of Liverpool, 1986.
2  Meissner DM. Porphyria in the Afrikaner population (letter). *South African Medical Journal* 1984; **65**: 277.
3  Cookson WO, Sharp PA, Faux JA, Hopkin JM. Linkage between immunoglobulin E responses underlying asthma and rhinitis and chromosome 11q. *Lancet* 1989; **i**: 1292–4.
4  Young RP, Sharp PA, Lynch JR, Faux JA, *et al*. Confirmation of genetic linkage between atopic IgE responses and chromosome 11q13. *Journal of Medical Genetics* 1992; **29**: 236–8.
5  Norton B. *A genetic study of Chester porphyria*. MD thesis, University of Liverpool, 1993.
6  Norton B, Lanyon WG, Moore MR, Porteous M, *et al*. Evidence for involvement of a second genetic locus on chromosome 11q in porphyrin metabolism. *Human Genetics* 1993; **91**: 576–8.
7  Cookson WOCM, Young RP, Sandford AJ, Moffat MF, *et al*. Maternal influence of atopic IgE responsiveness on chromosome 11q. *Lancet* 1992; **340**: 381–4.
8  Burr ML, Charles TJ, Roy K, Seaton A. Asthma in the elderly: an epidemiological survey. *British Medical Journal* 1979; **1**: 1041–4.
9  D'Souza MF. What factors are associated with reported asthma in middle age? *Clinical Allergy* 1979; **9**: 417–20.
10  Mullarkey MF, Thomas PS, Hansen JA, Webb DR, Nisperos B. Association of aspirin-sensitive asthma with HLA-DQw2. *American Review of Respiratory Disease* 1986; **133**: 261–3.
11  Slavin RG. Allergy is not a significant cause of nasal polyps (letter). *Archives of Otolaryngology – Head and Neck Surgery* 1992; **118**: 343.
12  Drake-Lee AA. Nasal polyps. In: Mackay IS (ed). *Rhinitis: mechanisms and management*. London: Royal Society of Medicine, 1989:141–52.
13  Keith PK, Conway M, Evans S, Wong DA, *et al*. Nasal polyps: effects of seasonal allergen exposure. *Journal of Allergy and Clinical Immunology* 1994; **93**: 567–74.

14 Durham SR, Kay AB. Eosinophils, bronchial hyperactivity and late-phase asthmatic reactions. *Clinical Allergy* 1985; **15**: 411–8.

15 Bentley AM, Menz G, Storz C, Robinson DS, *et al*. Identification of T lymphocytes, macrophages, and activated eosinophils in the bronchial mucosa in intrinsic asthma. Relationship to symptoms and bronchial responsiveness. *American Review of Respiratory Disease* 1992; **146**: 500–6.

16 Wong D, Jordana G, Denburg J, Dolovich J. Blood eosinophilia and nasal polyps. *American Journal of Rhinology* 1992; **6**: 195–8.

# Chapter 11

# Psychiatric morbidity in the kindred

ROGER CHITTY AND GILES YOUNGS

Many clinicians working in the field of porphyria have observed that psychiatric manifestations are common, but there is controversy as to whether they are temporary, arising only with a porphyric crisis, or whether there is a chronic disorder. It remains uncertain whether any psychiatric disturbance is directly due to a toxic effect of the excess raised porphyrin metabolites, a psychogenic response to illness, or the direct result of a mutation in the gene for porphobilinogen deaminase or a closely linked gene. Several recent observations implicate the long arm of chromosome 11 as a possible site for genes involved in the aetiology of schizophrenia and manic depression,[1,2] although other authors have failed to find an association between schizophrenia and porphobilinogen deaminase gene polymorphisms.[3–5]

## The Chester experience

Ten (21%) (nine porphyric, one (1.7) unknown status) of the 48 members of generations II and III of the Chester porphyria kindred have received inpatient care in the County Mental Hospital (Fig 1), at least four of them developing psychoses after barbiturate treatment (Table 1). The hospital had a large number of beds (reflecting its original catchment area of the whole of Cheshire), which may explain the apparent ease with which physicians and surgeons practising in the acute sector hospitals in the city seem to have been able to transfer their psychotic porphyria patients to psychiatric care. The number of psychiatric beds has now shrunk to one-thirteenth of the original complement (2,100 beds to 161), and transfer from the acute to the psychiatric sector requires the highest persuasive skills of the clinician in charge.

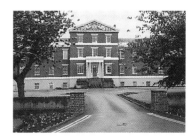

Fig 1. County Mental Hospital showing the Ionic porch and pediment of the '1829 Building' listed as a building of architectural and historical importance.

**Table 1.** Psychiatric morbidity in the Chester kindred.

| Notation | Gender | County Mental Hospital | Barbit-urates | Diagnosis | Notes |
|---|---|---|---|---|---|
| **Generation II** | | | | | |
| 1.5 | M | | + | Unknown | Strange manner |
| 1.6 | F | + | | Senile dementia | Anxiety neurosis |
| 1.7 | M | + | ? | Confusional insanity | Died age 36 in CMH after 3-year admission |
| 1.8 | F | + | ? | Unknown | Died age 32. Several admissions CMH |
| **Generation III** | | | | | |
| 1.2.1 | M | | ? | Mental deficiency | |
| 1.2.2 | M | | ? | Unknown | Strange character |
| 1.2.5 | F | | ? | Unknown | Reclusive |
| 1.2.8 | M | + | ? | Confusion | Died age 18, 12 days after leaving CMH |
| 1.5.1 | M | + | + | Depression | Attempted suicide |
| 1.5.2 | M | + | + | Acute psychosis | Post-operative |
| 1.5.3 | M | | + | Unknown | Odd personality. Drank vinegar |
| 1.6.3 | F | + | + | Acute psychosis | After treatment for malignant hypertension |
| 1.6.5 | M | | + | Hallucinations | |
| 1.8.1 | M | + | | Unknown | 4-year admission CMH |
| 1.8.2 | M | + | | Paranoid delusions | |
| 1.8.3 | F | + | | ?Acute psychosis | Given chlorpromazine |
| 1.9.2 | M | | | Agitation. Akathisia | Given chlorpromazine |
| 1.9.5 | F | | + | Acute psychosis | Post-operative |

CMH = County Mental Hospital.
? = no record of barbiturates, but psychiatric illness pre-1950 when these drugs were the mainstay of treatment.

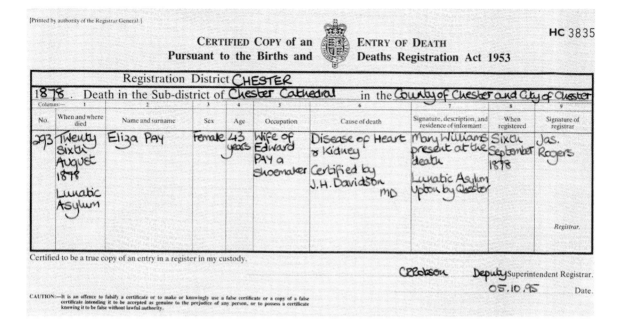

CERTIFIED COPY of an     ENTRY OF DEATH
Pursuant to the Births and     Deaths Registration Act 1953

HC 3835

Registration District CHESTER

18**78**.   Death in the Sub-district of Chester Cathedral   in the County of Chester and City of Chester

| No. | When and where died | Name and surname | Sex | Age | Occupation | Cause of death | Signature, description, and residence of informant | When registered | Signature of registrar |
|---|---|---|---|---|---|---|---|---|---|
| 293 | Twenty Sixth August 1878 Lunatic Asylum | Eliza Pay | Female | 43 years | Wife of Edward Pay a Shoemaker | Disease of Heart & Kidney Certified by J.H. Davidson MD | Mary Williams present at the death Lunatic Asylum Upton by Chester | Sixth September 1878 | Jas. Rogers |

Registrar.

Certified to be a true copy of an entry in a register in my custody.

C.P. Dobson    Deputy Superintendent Registrar.
    05.10.95    Date.

Fig 2. Eliza Pay's death certificate.

The Register of Admissions to the County Mental Hospital records that Eliza Pay, the mother of Sarah Pay, subsequently wife of Peter Dobson, the fisherman, was admitted in 1878 at the age of 43 with 'melancholia due to drink'. Diagnoses of other inpatients in this era were equally picturesque, and included 'disappointment in love', 'religious excitement', 'fright from a dream' and, more prosaically, 'loss of money'. This proved to be Eliza Pay's terminal illness – she died in the lunatic asylum of disease of the heart and kidneys (Fig 2).

## Psychiatric history in generations I and II

*1.5*: an obligatory porphyric, died age 83 in 1980 in a psychogeriatric ward at the County Mental Hospital. Ten years earlier he had been admitted to Chester Royal Infirmary for a cataract operation, and was given butobarbitone 100 mg each night. He had a very strange manner and was difficult at times; he would not talk to the other patients, and refused his porridge.

*1.6*: his sister, died age 81 in 1982 in a psychogeriatric ward at the County Mental Hospital. She was the only member of this generation that one of us (GRY) met. She had no recorded porphyric symptoms but had 'anxiety neurosis' throughout her life. In 1967, she had a laparotomy for bleeding gastric ulcer. She seems not to have been upset by the perhaps customary night sedation of amylobarbitone sodium and then butobarbitone.

153

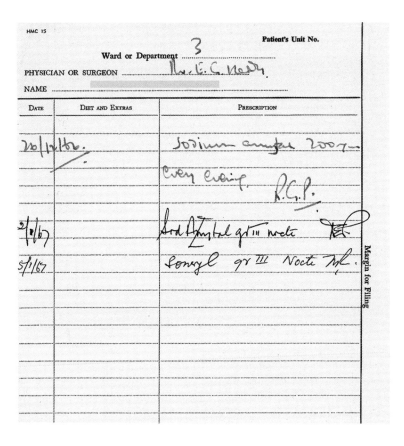

**Fig 3**. Drug prescription chart (1967) of subject 1.6 showing barbiturate prescriptions written in both apothecaries' and metric notation.

These prescriptions (Fig 3) were made at the time of change over from apothecaries' to metric drug dosages. Her first prescription for sodium amytal 200 mg every evening was rewritten a week later as sodium amytal grains iii nocte. On 3rd March 1969, it became illegal to use any system of weights and measures other than the metric system for dispensing (but not for prescribing) drugs.[6]

Her daughter *1.6.3* (Chapter 4), son *1.6.5* (Chapters 6 and 7) and grandson *1.6.5.1* (Chapter 6) died of porphyria; her granddaughter, *1.6.5.3*, was the teenager met in outpatients in 1980 (Chapters 1 and 7).

*1.7*: her brother, a labourer, died age 36 in 1940 in the County Mental Hospital of influenzal pneumonia. His hospital case-sheet records that he was admitted with the diagnosis of confusional insanity. 'His train of thought is incoherent and he believes he hears voices.' His wife reported a history of severe pains in the head. The case-notes are incomplete, and there is no record of abdominal pain, dark urine or any medication prescribed. Three days before his death he developed persistent vomiting and diarrhoea.

*1.7.2* and *1.7.3*: two of his three children, have been tested for porphyria and are negative.

154

*1.7.1*: his third child, died after an appendix operation in Australia, age 31 years. Bekerus felt that porphyria was implicated in this case. Qadiri was told he had paralysis, but two of his three children have been tested for porphyria in Australia with negative results. Thus, subject 1.7 is of unknown porphyria status.

*1.8*: sister of 1.7, is said by her family to have had admissions to the County Mental Hospital with delirium. She died age 31 in 1938 in Chester City Hospital of lobar pneumonia. She is an obligatory carrier of porphyria.

## Psychiatric history in generation III

The psychiatric problems in the 38 grandchildren are better documented:

*1.2.1*: died age 29 in 1946 of uraemia, nephritis and mental deficiency. No further details are known, except that Bekerus was told he was 'mentally affected'.

*1.2.2*: his brother, was a 'strange character with long finger-nails'.

*1.2.5*: their sister, was reclusive.

*1.2.8*: another brother, died age 18 years in 1953. He became paralysed and confused (according to Bekerus), and became a voluntary patient in the County Mental Hospital. Only brief details are available, and medication is not recorded. He died 12 days after discharge. His death certificate records left ventricular failure and malignant hypertension.

None of these four siblings had children, but on circumstantial evidence we believe that 1.2.1 and 1.2.8 were both porphyric (Chapter 6), and that the status of 1.2.2 and 1.2.5 is unknown.

*1.5.1*: their cousin, died age 60 in 1981. He had a history of headaches, depression and several suicide attempts. He was in the County Mental Hospital in 1963 when Bekerus found his urine first negative for porphobilinogen 'until the general practitioner (GP) loaded him with barbiturates'. Subsequently, he had a course of electroconvulsive therapy. He was divorced from his first wife in 1968; she recalls severe bouts of temper and blackouts. He died in Chester City Hospital after living for some time in a hostel.

*1.5.2*: his brother, died age 67 in 1988. He was admitted to Chester Royal Infirmary in 1964 with a history of severe epigastric pain and vomiting. The referring GP opined that 'undoubtedly he must have a penetrating peptic ulcer', and mentioned that the patient's brother (1.5.3) had died in Chester City Hospital 10 years previously of peripheral neuritis after being admitted with 'peptic ulcer'. The patient was prescribed propantheline and, for no obvious reason – other than a possible perceived role for sedation in peptic ulcer – also barbiturates on 9th and

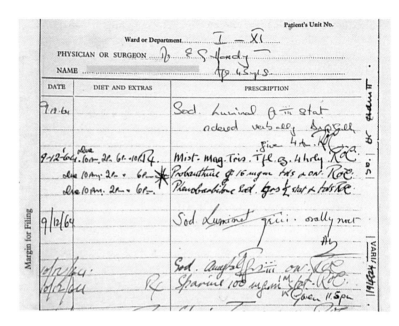

**Fig 4.** Drug prescription chart (1964) of subject 1.5.2 showing barbiturate prescriptions.

10th December 1964 (Fig 4). On 12th December the consultant surgeon, Mr EG Hardy, recorded:

> A very odd chap. I think the trouble may be functional but I don't want to do him an injustice. For barium meal. If negative I think we might ask Dr Dewi Jones to see him.

This psychiatric consultation duly followed:

> Clearly psychotic, and has been put on a Section 25 and to be admitted to Deva (County Mental Hospital) today.

Meanwhile a barium meal was normal. On the night of his admission to the mental hospital he was given sodium amytal grains 6, and he became both mentally and physically worse. A message then came through that a cousin was known to have porphyria – and, indeed, urine testing for porphobilinogen on 1.5.2 was positive. When he became mentally normal, an EEG was performed after giving him phenobarbitone grains ½ as an aid to interpretation. He again became briefly mentally confused. During his four-week admission, he developed marked weakness of the right arm and his calf muscles appeared 'rather flabby'. A subsequent letter from his GP in 1976 refers to the sobriquet 'Dobson's complaint' (Fig 8, Chapter 1). Ironically, he died in 1988 two days after a massive haemorrhage from a gastric ulcer requiring urgent partial gastrectomy.

**1.5.3**: his brother, a driver salesman of an ice cream van, died age 30 in 1953 of pneumonia, paralysis and peripheral neuritis after being admitted with abdominal pain thought to be due to peptic ulcer. He had an odd personality and used to drink vinegar. Bekerus records that he was treated with barbiturates. He is an obligatory carrier of porphyria.

156

*1.5.5*: a fourth brother, died age 51 in 1982. His story is recorded in Chapter 6. He became depressed and developed hallucinations. He was admitted to the County Mental Hospital in 1981 after being found at home lying on the floor, conscious but neglected. He was treated with tricyclic antidepressants, and began to hear voices commanding him to clean the toilets. He developed bizarre behaviour, licking urine from the floor. Subsequently, he developed an epileptic fit, meningism then coma, but serum electrolytes remained normal and he was normotensive. Necropsy failed to reveal the cause of death, but we feel this was a porphyric death precipitated by tricyclic antidepressant therapy. He is an obligatory carrier of porphyria.

*1.6.3*: wife of a gas fitter, died age 46 in 1978 of cerebellar haemorrhage. Her admission to the County Mental Hospital with an acute psychosis after treatment (probably with barbiturates) for malignant hypertension is the subject of Chapter 4. Her EEG was grossly abnormal.

*1.6.5*: her brother, had an epileptic fit in the army and was treated with barbiturates which caused a porphyric crisis (Chapter 6). He was admitted with a further crisis two months later, and developed hallucinations and neuropathy. His EEG was grossly abnormal.

*1.8.1*: aged 67, was admitted to the County Mental Hospital at the age of 40, where he remained under psychiatric care for four years.

*1.8.2*: his brother aged 62, had an admission to the County Mental Hospital in 1973 at the age of 39 because of paranoid delusions. He initially required regular sedation with chlorpromazine. The consultant psychiatrist, Dr KCS Edwards wrote to the GP:

> *Whether this episode was due to porphyria I don't really know, although one does see patients with this condition who do suffer from mood changes, although in his case it does not seem to have been associated with confusion and headache, which is so often the case.*

*1.8.3*: their sister, died age 47 in 1982 of renal failure and acute intermittent porphyria. Bekerus records that in the winter she took sleeping tablets and developed 'gastric sickness', constipation, backache, headache and red urine positive for porphobilinogen. She was admitted in 1982 with severe renal failure (Chapter 8), and required chlorpromazine (presumably for acute psychosis).

*1.9.2*: a labourer (Chapter 8), died age 55 in 1988 of chronic renal failure and hypertension. He developed asthma on propranolol, which was replaced with indoramin. He became rather agitated, and in 1981 was given chlorpromazine 100 mg nocte for a year. He developed several extrapyramidal features (tremor, tardive dyskinesia and disabling akathisia) which persisted. In 1986, he developed a severe peripheral neuropathy for which he was in hospital six months.

*1.9.5*: his sister, developed a severe psychiatric disturbance and then coma after an anaesthetic was given for sterilisation in the Chester City

Hospital in 1971 – despite her reporting that she had positive tests for porphyria (with Bekerus) a few years before. The story is corroborated by the consultant physician who subsequently advised. Her husband refused permission for transfer to the County Mental Hospital.

In more recent times, acute porphyric crises in our subjects, particularly 1.6.5.3 (Chapter 7) and 1.8.3.3 (Chapter 6), have invariably been associated with misery and distress, but not frank psychosis. The general anguish of the attack, interspersed with frequent pleas for analgesia, often leads to suspicions of hysteria, as noted in subjects 1.6.3 (Chapter 4) and also 1.6.5.1 (Chapter 6) who was given an injection of sterile water the day before he died age 17. The senior great-grandchild, 1.1.1.1, a clerk at the Countess of Chester Hospital, vividly remembers being suspected of hysteria by both nursing and surgical staff when admitted in 1962 at the age of 22 to the Chester Royal Infirmary as a surgical emergency with abdominal and generalised body pain. It was suggested that her symptoms were related to the television programme 'Emergency Ward 10'. She was given barbiturates during convalescence. Our two subjects 1.6.5.3 and 1.8.3.3 occasionally developed confusion and hallucinations coincident with hyponatraemia (Chapter 9). Unfortunately, we have no information about electrolytes (except that they were normal in 1.5.5) in the many cases of florid psychosis in the senior family members described earlier in the chapter.

In summary, some of our family members were misdiagnosed as suffering from pure psychiatric conditions and admitted to psychiatric wards (eg brothers 1.5.1, 1.5.5) or transferred to the psychiatric hospital because of acute psychosis complicating apparent organic illnesses (eg 1.5.2, 1.6.3). We know that two subjects (1.5.2, 1.9.5) developed acute psychoses after a barbiturate anaesthetic, and two (1.6.3, 1.6.5) did so after barbiturates for malignant hypertension and epilepsy, respectively. We believe that the psychosis and subsequent death in 1.5.5 were due to porphyric complications of tricyclic antidepressant administration. The onset of akathisia in 1.9.2 coincided with indoramin treatment, and worsened when chlorpromazine was prescribed for the agitation.

Eight of the 38 grandchildren with psychiatric morbidity are known to have had treatment with barbiturates, and six had admissions to the County Mental Hospital. We strongly suspect that six others in generations II and III (1.7, 1.9, 1.2.1, 1.2.2, 1.2.5, 1.2.8) may also have received this ubiquitous medication from the 1940s onwards.

In contrast, although 43 (27%) of 158 porphyric patients in Finland[7] described neuropsychiatric symptoms, only three received psychiatric care. In fact, the age- and sex-specific prevalence rates of neuropsychiatric symptoms among the subjects with porphyria were not significantly higher than in the general Finnish population, except among women with porphyria aged 30–44 years.

Happily, it is many years since a Chester family member received inpatient psychiatric care. We believe that our data show that serious and chronic psychiatric morbidity in our family largely occurred in the barbiturate era, and therefore afflicted the children and grandchildren of Peter and Sarah Dobson but not the next generation. Regrettably, many family members are ashamed of this history of psychiatric illness in themselves and their kin. Some have denied that the taint of porphyria affects their branch of the family, which may explain why some have declined to participate in the family study. Similar shame is reported in Arjeplog, northern Sweden.[8]

It is intriguing that Eliza Pay, the maternal grandmother of the 10 siblings, died in the County Mental Hospital age 43 with disease of the heart and kidneys (Fig 2), having been admitted with melancholia due to drink. Many of her offspring died of malignant hypertension and renal failure, raising the possibility that they inherited these tendencies, and perhaps the causative porphyria, from Eliza. On the other hand, there is circumstantial evidence that the porphyria came from the paternal side (Chapter 3).

## Is the psychiatric abnormality inborn, toxic or a psychogenic response to illness?

It is 60 years since Waldenström[9,10] reported that many of his porphyric patients in northern Sweden had been sent to an asylum, and that some developed the syndrome of acute psychosis with polyneuritis epitomised by our subject 1.6.3 (Chapter 4). His family study showed that schizophrenia and manic depressive illness appeared to be common in porphyric families, although no statistical analysis was given. Wetterberg[11] subsequently re-examined these families, and suggested independent inheritance of acute intermittent porphyria and mental illness. He introduced the term 'acute intermittent porphyria mental syndrome', which he regarded as an organic brain disturbance due to porphyria. (Some of the mechanisms which may explain disturbed cerebral function are discussed in Chapter 7.)

Goldberg[12] found that 29 (58%) of 50 consecutive cases of porphyria admitted to hospital had mental symptoms (depression, nervousness or hysterical, lachrymose or 'peculiar' behaviour: 14; confusion, disorientation, hallucinations or personality change: 9; 'legally certified': 6). Patience et al[13] extended this series, and found 16 patients with 'psychiatric contact' in 344 consecutive patients admitted to the Western Infirmary, Glasgow. Family members of 12 of the 16 were studied using structured questionnaires, but no association was found between acute intermittent porphyria and schizophrenia or manic depressive illness. The commonest psychiatric diagnosis was generalised anxiety, which correlated with the level of porphyrin metabolites in the urine at the time of assessment, even in subjects with latent porphyria.

This, however, contrasted with the finding by Ackner et al[14] of no correlation between psychiatric symptoms and excretion in the urine of delta-aminolaevulinic acid. In their study of 13 patients, all but one had essentially normal personalities. Similarly, Luby et al[15] found no consistent pattern using the Minnesota Multiphasic Personality Inventory, and Wetterberg and Österberg[16] found no difference from controls with the Maudsley Personality Inventory in 25 cases of acute intermittent porphyria. Dean and Barnes[17] failed to show an increased prevalence of porphyria variegata in South African mental hospitals.

These studies suggest that psychiatric symptoms in subjects with porphyria are usually fairly mild, or at least short-lived. Several other surveys, however, have described an increased prevalence of acute intermittent porphyria in psychiatric hospitals, which hints at more chronic and serious psychiatric morbidity.[18-20] The DSM-III diagnoses of the patients in the last study[20] were atypical psychosis and schizoaffective disorder. Thus, porphyria may be overlooked in the assessment of patients with puzzling neuropsychiatric symptoms.[21]

There have even been claims that mental disorder underlies and causes attacks of acute porphyria. Roth[22] found that porphyria occurred with special frequency, if not exclusively, amongst people with severe neurotic personality disorders. The patients usually appeared to be hysterical, except those in whom organic brain disease clouded the underlying features of their personality. He thought it probable that psychoneurosis played a large part both in the pathogenesis of the disease and in determining the time of the acute attack. He also noted that porphyria occurred in families in which psychiatric disorders were rife.

Kark[23] suggested a more chronic personality disorder, which he termed 'termagantism'. He wrote:

*Bedevilled as they are by their disease, the victims of porphyria go from doctor to doctor seeking a diagnosis – if one is not made – or a cure for their disorder. They are resentful, irascible, unpredictable, vituperative, violent in temper, and liable to burst into tears or a tantrum at a moment's notice. In this respect they remind one of Katherine, the virago of Shakespeare's* Taming of the Shrew. *To call attention to this mental agitation, which may persist in remissions from the disease long after other signs and symptoms have disappeared, I have coined the term 'termagantism'. The word 'termagant', which is still in common usage, is quite an old one. It is derived from the Mohammedan word for 'devil', usually a woman of turbulent character, who appeared in medieval morality plays.*

*When muscle pain or colic is continuous or severe, patients with porphyria become peevish and whining, their voice develops a high pitched nasal quality and they constantly complain in a 'neurotic' way. This seemingly unreasonable behavior pattern forces the label of 'hysteria' on them, especially when the diagnosis is not at hand. In the cases we have seen in consultation, 'hysteria' was the most common diagnosis made by the family physician. But their behavior is not hysterical. Most patients with hysterical complaints, such as anorexia nervosa, globus hystericus, pseudocyesis and hysterical paralysis, are not resentful. Their personality pattern is often a passive one. They 'accept' their infirmities. When they make a scene to draw attention to themselves it is soon over, and separated from the next tantrum by acceptable behaviour.*

*The vicious acerbity of the conduct of porphyrinuric termagants makes it difficult at times to treat them on a medical ward. Nurses dislike caring for them. They are a troublesome group of patients and kindle feelings of hatred and aggression in the most urbane physicians. A very gentle psychiatrist, talking of one patient we were looking after, remarked 'Her husband must be an angel. How he lives with her I do not know. I think I would have done away with her long ago'.*

Kark's graphic prose captures some of the exasperation echoed in the medical and nursing notes of our hapless family members, but how galling it must have been for subject 1.6.3 (Chapter 4) to have been suspected of hysteria when she lay in bed in the County Mental Hospital unable to adjust her position because of a complete flaccid paralysis. Even today, 25 years later, the family of subject 1.9.1 remain indignant that, despite their warnings, she received a thiopentone anaesthesia, which resulted in an acute psychosis for which transfer to the mental hospital was planned but which her husband refused.

We can only speculate whether any element of termagantism in our family explains the tumultuous behaviour of the fisher-folk in Stye Lane, so well recorded over the decades in the Chester Chronicle (Chapter 3).

## A psychometric study of the Chester kindred

Because of the degree of mental illness exhibited by sufferers of Chester porphyria and the controversy whether such disorders are acute or chronic, we decided to study the association between psychiatric disorder and porphyria within the family. Ethical committee approval was obtained.

*The General Health Questionnaire 60*

For this study, we chose the General Health Questionnaire (GHQ) 60,[24] a self-administered screening test which detects psychiatric disorder in community and non-psychiatric clinical settings, and which has been found acceptable to respondents. It gives an estimate of the probability of an individual being a psychiatric 'case', although it does not provide a diagnosis. It focuses on breaks in normal functioning (ie the ability to perform normal functions) and on new, distressing phenomena. It is not designed to estimate personality disorder, mental handicap or psychotic disorder. It can be used to detect hidden psychiatric disorder in the population in a categorical (case vs non-case) or dimensional way, the score of an individual being a rough proxy measure of the position of that individual on a hypothetical underlying dimension of psychiatric illness. This does not require the respondent to be characterised either as a case or a non-case and the dimensional scores can be compared between groups of subjects without assumptions being made about an individual's psychiatric 'caseness'.

High scores suggest psychiatric disorder, some authors using a score of 12 to separate normals from abnormals. Additionally, the data from the GHQ60 can be subdivided in two ways:

- A subset of 28 questions (GHQ28) yields four subscales:
  - somatic symptoms,
  - social dysfunction,
  - severe depression, and
  - anxiety and insomnia.
- A different subset of 30 questions (CGHQ)[25,26] indicates chronicity of any psychiatric disturbance.

*Patients and methods*

Sixty-seven subjects age 16 years and over were identified from the Chester porphyria register. None of the 32 who had porphyria was known to be in porphyric crisis at the time of the study. The remainder without porphyria were first-degree relatives of those with porphyria. A questionnaire was sent to all of them, together with a letter of explanation and a stamped addressed envelope in which to return the completed questionnaire. A second questionnaire and letter of reminder were sent one month later to those people who had not responded. The scores were compared between:

- the porphyria-negative (control group) and porphyria-positive subjects;
- the control group and latent porphyrics;
- the control group and symptomatic porphyrics; and

- the scores, weighted according to gender, and those of a standard 'English' population mean quoted by Goldberg.[24]

The data from the GHQ60 and CGHQ were used to compare the control with the porphyria groups.

## Statistical analysis

The comparisons of the data were analysed using Student's $t$-test (two-tailed) and $\chi$-squared statistics. Although both statistical methods may be employed,[25] the latter is more appropriate if the data are not randomly distributed.

## Results

Seventeen of the 32 porphyria-positive subjects (53%) returned the questionnaire, 16 (50%) of which were suitable for analysis. The average age of the respondents was 37 years (range 17–63 years), six had symptomatic porphyria and 10 were latent porphyrics. Sixteen of the 35 non-porphyric family members (46%) returned the questionnaire. Their average age was 34 years (range 18–66 years). Each group of 16 subjects contained nine males.

There was no significant difference between the mean GHQ60 scores for the control and porphyria groups, nor a significant sex difference (Table 2). A $\chi$-squared table, which was constructed (Table 3) because of the large standard deviations, also showed no significant difference between the groups. There was no measurable difference between porphyrics and non-porphyrics when the GHQ28 subscales were employed, and their scores were similar using the subset (CGHQ) which measures chronicity of psychiatric disorder (Table 2).

Table 2. General Health Questionnaire (GHQ) 60 and GHQ measuring chronicity (CGHQ): scores in porphyric and non-porphyric family members.

| | Non-porphyria | Porphyria | | | All male | All female | Standard 'English' population |
| | | Symptomatic | Latent | All | | | |
| --- | --- | --- | --- | --- | --- | --- | --- |
| No. | 16 | 6 | 10 | 16 | 18 | 14 | |
| GHQ60 mean score (range) | 7.3 (0–41) | 7.3 (0–22) | 13.9 (0–47) | 11.4 (0–47) | 11.6 (0–47) | 6.4 (0–22) | 9.0 |
| CGHQ mean score (range) | 8.1 (0–22) | 7.8 (2–16) | 11.0 (1–28) | 9.8 (1–28) | 9.7 (1–28) | 8.1 (0–22) | |

GHQ60: comparing non-porphyria (standard deviation (SD): 10.7) with all porphyria (SD: 13.1): $t = 0.97$, $p = 0.341$. Not significant.
CGHQ: comparing non-porphyria (SD: 6.6) with all porphyria (SD: 7.7): $t = 0.66$, $p = 0.513$. Not significant.

**Table 3.** General Health Questionnaire 60: porphyric and non-porphyric members with low and high scores ($\chi$-squared).

| | Score | | | |
|---|---|---|---|---|
| | Less than 12 | | 12 or above | |
| | No. | % | No. | % |
| Porphyria | 10 | 63 | 6 | 37 |
| Non-porphyria | 13 | 82 | 3 | 18 |
| Total | 23 | | 9 | |

$\chi^2 = 0.6184$. Not significant.

## Discussion

The psychometric study was designed to find out if psychiatric disorder is more common in the porphyric than non-porphyric members of the kindred. The strength of the study is that it was performed within the kindred so that the controls came from a similar social and genetic background rather than from an arbitrary source. The weakness of the study is the inevitable small numbers of subjects recruited, although the response rate of 50% was good (Brodie et al[27] report a 10–57% range of response rates to postal surveys).

No significant difference was found between the study groups. This is, of course, not the same as saying that psychiatric disturbance is therefore *equal* in porphyric and non-porphyric subjects, but the scores for chronic psychiatric disturbance were very *similar*. Unlike Patience et al,[13] no difference was found in chronic anxiety measured by GHQ28 between the two groups. Andersson, in Arjeplog, found only small psychosocial differences in porphyric subjects compared to controls sent a questionnaire.[8]

There can be no doubt that psychiatric illness was unusually common in the porphyric members of the family (Table 1). We know of no non-porphyric members who had psychiatric illness or admission to the County Mental Hospital, despite a search of the hospital's archives for the name Dobson. Bekerus discovered that the cousins admitted to that hospital in the 1960s received barbiturates. Fortunately, no family member has needed psychiatric admission since subject 1.5.5's pre-terminal admission in 1981.

Moore and Hift[28] suggest that the acute hepatic porphyrias are examples of 'toxico-genetic diseases'. This seems reasonable, but should not imply that the disease is manifest only if the subject is exposed to drugs or toxins. The label 'ecogenic disorder', suggested by Desnick's group,[29] may be preferable since the expression of porphyria is often precipitated by hormonal, metabolic, dietary or environmental factors. Our two young female subjects (1.6.5.3, 1.8.3.3) received no drugs before their 31 admissions, but their attacks were often premenstrual (Chapter 7). They were both distressed and emotionally upset, crying out, withdrawn, and frequently pleading for opiates. The appellation 'toxico-genetic' applies well, however, to the psychotic manifestations of porphyria, and we feel sure that the serious psychiatric illness and subsequent death of many subjects were iatrogenic. Our experience is neatly echoed by Tschudy:[30]

> We have seen psychiatric symptoms develop in patients given pentothal for dental proceedings – only to receive barbiturates again to control those psychiatric symptoms.

Our psychometric study suggests that if drugs are avoided, psychiatric 'caseness' is equal in porphyric and non-porphyric family members when the former are not in porphyric crisis.

Clinicians should heed Waldenström's warning about misdiagnosing hysteria.[10,31] Despite our experience of porphyric crises in the Chester family, and although we still find the emotional aspects of the illness difficult to assess, we do not go as far as Kark[23] in his belief of a chronic state of termagantism.

# References

1 Grandy DK, Litt M, Allen L, Bunzow JR, *et al*. The human dopamine D2 receptor gene is located on chromosome 11 at q22–q23 and identifies a Taq1 RFLP. *American Journal of Human Genetics* 1989; **45**: 778–85.

2 Sanders AR, Rincon-Limas DE, Chakraborty R, Grandchamp B, *et al*. Association between genetic variation at the porphobilinogen deaminase gene with schizophrenia. *Schizophrenia Research* 1993; **8**: 211–21.

3 Nimgaonkar VL, Ganguli R, Washington SS, Chakravarti A. Schizophrenia and porphobilinogen deaminase gene polymorphisms: an association study. *Schizophrenia Research* 1992; **8**: 51-8.

4 Gill M, McGuffin P, Parfitt E, Mant R, *et al*. A linkage study of schizophrenia with DNA markers from the long arm of chromosome 11. *Psychological Medicine* 1993; **23**: 27–44.

5 Wang ZW, Black D, Andreasen NC, Crowe RR. A linkage study of chromosome 11q in schizophrenia. *Archives of General Psychiatry* 1993; **50**: 212–6.

6 Changeover to metric. *Pharmaceutical Journal* 1969; **202**: 231–8.

7 Kauppinen R, Mustajoki P. Prognosis of acute porphyria: occurrence of acute attacks, precipitating factors, and associated diseases. *Medicine* 1992; **71**: 1–13.

8  Andersson C, Gåfvels C, Lithner F. Living with acute intermittent porphyria. A socio-medical study in northern Sweden. In: Andersson C
   (ed). *Acute intermittent porphyria in Northern Sweden: a population-
   based study*. Umeå University Medical Dissertations, New Series
   No. 497. Umeå and Arjeplog, Sweden: University of Umeå and Primary Health Care Centre, Arjeplog, 1997. (Also submitted for separate
   publication.)

9  Waldenström J. Studien über porphyrie. *Acta Medica Scandinavica*
   1937; **92** (Suppl 82): 1–254.

10 Waldenström J. Neurological symptoms caused by so called acute porphyria. *Acta Psychiatrica et Neurologica* 1939; **14**: 375–9.

11 Wetterberg L. *A neuropsychiatric and genetical investigation of acute
   intermittent porphyria*. Stockholm: Svenska Bokforlaget, 1967.

12 Goldberg A. Acute intermittent porphyria. A study of 50 cases. *Quarterly Journal of Medicine* 1959; **NS28**: 183–209.

13 Patience DA, Blackwood DHR, McColl KEL, Moore MR. Acute intermittent porphyria and mental illness – a family study. *Acta Psychiatrica
   Scandinavica* 1994; **89**: 262–7.

14 Ackner B, Cooper JE, Gray CH, Kelly M. Acute porphyria: a neuropsychiatric and biochemical study. *Journal of Psychosomatic Research*
   1962; **6**: 1–24.

15 Luby ED, Ware JG, Senf R, Frohman CE. Stress and the precipitation
   of acute intermittent porphyria. *Psychosomatic Medicine* 1959; **21**:
   34–49.

16 Wetterberg L, Österberg E. Acute intermittent porphyria: a psychometric study of twenty-five patients. *Journal of Psychosomatic Research*
   1970; **13**: 91–3.

17 Dean G, Barnes HD. Porphyria: a South African screening experiment.
   *British Medical Journal* 1958; **1**: 298–301.

18 Kaelbling R, Craig JB, Pasamanick B. Urinary porphobilinogen. Results
   of screening 2,500 psychiatric patients. *Archives of General Psychiatry*
   1961; **5**: 494–508.

19 McEwin R, Lawn J, Jonas CT. A survey of porphyria among psychiatric patients. *Medical Journal of Australia* 1972; **2**: 303–6.

20 Tishler PV, Woodward B, O'Connor J, Holbrook DA, *et al.* High prevalence of intermittent acute porphyria in a psychiatric patient population. *American Journal of Psychiatry* 1985; **142**: 1430–6.

21 Crimlisk HL. The little imitator – porphyria: a neuropsychiatric disorder. *Journal of Neurology, Neurosurgery and Psychiatry* 1997; **62**:
   319–28.

22 Roth N. The neuropsychiatric aspects of porphyria. *Psychosomatic
   Medicine* 1945; **7**: 291–301.

23 Kark RM. Clinical aspects of the major porphyrinopathies. *Medical
   Clinics of North America* 1955; **39**: 11–30.

24 Goldberg DP. *The detection of psychiatric illness by questionnaire*.
   Maudsley Monograph No. 21. Oxford: Oxford University Press, 1972.

25 Goldberg DP, Williams P. *A user's guide to the General Health Questionnaire*. Windsor: NFER-Nelson Publishing Company, 1988.

26 Goodchild ME, Duncan-Jones P. Chronicity and the General Health Questionnaire. *British Journal of Psychiatry* 1985; **146**: 55–61.

27 Brodie DA, Williams JG, Owens RG. *Research methods for the health sciences*. Chur, Switzerland: Harwood Academic Publishers, 1994.

28 Moore MR, Hift RJ. Drugs in the acute porphyrias – toxicogenetic diseases. *Cellular and Molecular Biology* 1997; **43**: 89–94.

29 McGovern MM, Anderson KE, Astrin KH, Desnick RJ. Inherited porphyrias. In: Emery A (ed). *Principles and practice of medical genetics*. Edinburgh: Churchill Livingstone, 1996: 2009–36

30 Tschudy DP, Valsamis M, Magnussen CR. Acute intermittent porphyria: clinical and selected research aspects. *Annals of Internal Medicine* 1975; **83**: 851–64

31 Waldenström J. The porphyrias as inborn errors of metabolism. *American Journal of Medicine* 1957; **22**: 758–73.

# Chapter 12

# The biochemistry of Chester porphyria

MICHAEL MOORE

## Part 1: Porphyrins and the porphyrias

### Porphyrins

Porphyrins are fascinating compounds. In the biosphere, they are used most effectively in the process of energy capture and utilisation.[1] Abiotic formation of porphyrins, in particular of uroporphyrinogen, would probably have provided the first of the pigments necessary for the eventual synthesis of the chlorophylls,[2] thereby facilitating the emergence of simple photosynthetic organisms on primordial earth through enhanced efficiency of energy capture. In living organisms, the porphyrins exist in the reduced hexahydro form, the porphyrinogen. The structure of protoporphyrinogen (PROTO), the compound of greatest importance in Chester porphyria, is shown in Fig 1.

From the outset, the name 'porphyria' described not the diseases but the lustrous purple-red crystalline porphyrins named from the Greek *porfuros* (*porphuros* or purple). The normal biological intermediate is not this highly conjugated porphyrin, but the hexahydroporphyrin. An important feature of this complex ring structure is its metal-binding capability. The commonest metals bound are iron and magnesium. In these bound forms, namely, haem and chlorophylls, the metalloporphyrins reach their true apotheosis:

- *Haem*, the iron-containing complex, usually bound to various proteins, is central to all biological oxidations and to oxygen transport.
- *Chlorophylls*, the magnesium-porphyrin compounds, are pivotal in solar energy utilisation in the biosphere.

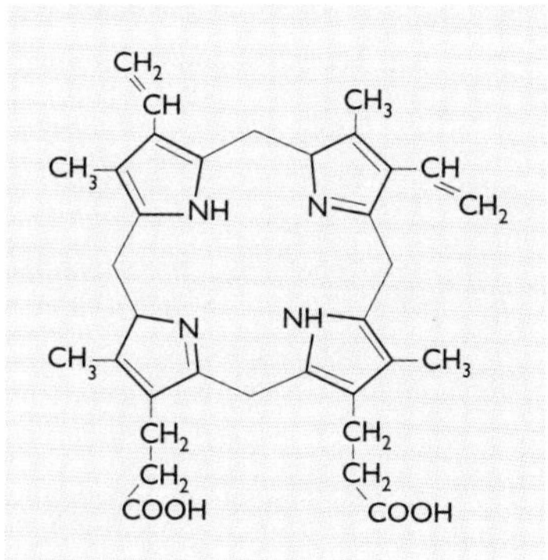

Fig 1. Molecular structure of protoporphyrinogen.

Porphyrins are also used in pigmentation, such as in turacin, the copper-uroporphyrin III complex which colours the feathers of the Cape Lowry[3] or provides the pigmentation of eggshells.[4] The Nobel laureate, Hans Fischer, described them as the compounds that make grass green and blood red.

## The porphyrias

The porphyrias are inherited disorders of haem biosynthesis in which specific abnormalities of enzymes in the haem biosynthetic pathway cause generalised clinical abnormalities. The florid clinical picture can be precipitated by drugs, hormonal factors and ethanol consumption. They may be classified into acute and non-acute porphyrias (Table 1).

All the porphyrias are inherited as autosomal dominant traits, except for the rare congenital form, which is recessive, and the few cases observed to date of homozygous inheritance of a number of the porphyrias.[5,6] Many studies of families with acute hepatic porphyria show that only a small proportion of gene carriers have symptomatic disease,[7] although this is not true either in generation III of the Chester family (Chapter 7) or in a recent survey of subjects with acute intermittent porphyria in a Swedish municipality.[8,9] Examples of controversial retrospective studies of the possible presence of acute porphyria include those of the British Royal Family[10,11] and the family of Vincent van Gogh.[12] The best demonstration is of variegate porphyria in South Africa.[13] The incidence of new mutations is difficult to estimate: it has been suggested that they occur in 3% of acute intermittent porphyria cases.[14]

There is a reduction of gene frequency from generation to generation, suggesting that the allele associated with variegate

Table 1. Classification of the porphyrias.

| | Type of porphyria | Synonym |
|---|---|---|
| Acute | Acute intermittent porphyria | Swedish porphyria |
| | Variegate porphyria | South African genetic porphyria |
| | Hereditary coproporphyria | Coproporphyria |
| | Plumboporphyria | ALA dehydratase deficiency porphyria |
| Non-acute | Congenital porphyria | Günther's disease |
| | Porphyria cutanea tarda | Cutaneous hepatic porphyria; symptomatic porphyria |
| | Erythropoietic protoporphyria | Erythrohepatic porphyria |

ALA= delta-aminolaevulinic acid

porphyria is selectively deleterious.[15] The same is probably true of the other porphyrias: in the Chester family, six cousins (Table 1, Chapter 7) and two members of the succeeding generation (Chapter 7) died from porphyria age 30 years or less.

## Haem biosynthesis

Each of the different types of porphyria is linked to a deficiency in a specific enzyme in the haem biosynthetic pathway (Figs 2 and 3); in some circumstances, more than one enzyme may be affected. As a result of the enzyme block in haem synthesis, there is a compensatory increase in the activity of the initial and rate-controlling enzyme of the pathway, delta-aminolaevulinic acid (ALA) synthase, and by overproduction of the porphyrins and their precursors formed before the enzyme block. This enzyme is under negative feedback control by haem. Attacks of neurovisceral dysfunction associated with overproduction of the porphyrin precursors, ALA and porphobilinogen (PBG) are common in all the acute porphyrias.

Fig 2. Diagrammatic representation of haem biosynthesis:
ALA = delta-aminolaevulinic acid;
CoA = coenzyme A;
Copro = coproporphyrin;
Fe = iron;
PBG = porphobilinogen;
PROTO = protoporphyrinogen;
Uro = uroporphyrinogen.

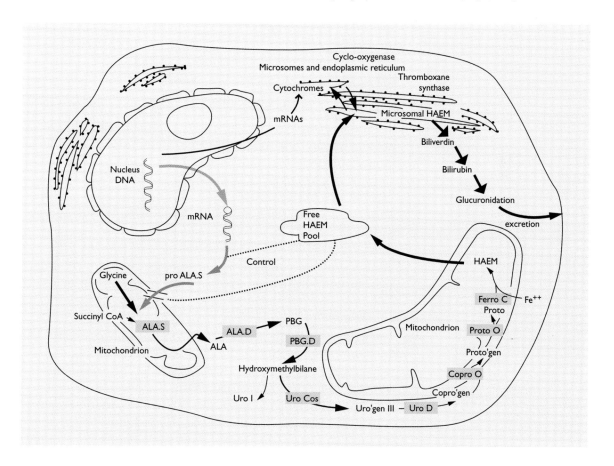

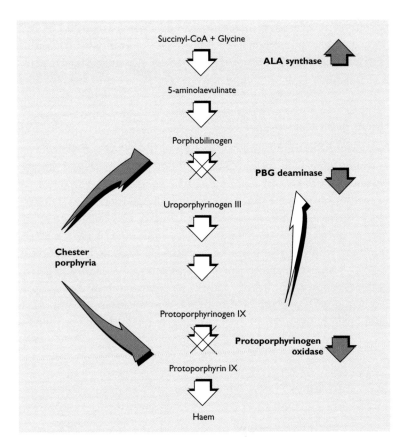

**Fig 3.** Haem biosynthesis in Chester porphyria:
ALA = delta-aminolaevulinic acid;
CoA = coenzyme A;
PBG = porphobilinogen.

In variegate porphyria and hereditary coproporphyria, cutaneous photosensitivity also occurs because of the overproduction of formed porphyrins.

*Acute intermittent porphyria*

The activity of the third enzyme of the pathway, PBG deaminase, is reduced by 50% in acute intermittent porphyria,[16] resulting in various degrees of overproduction and increased urinary excretion of ALA and PBG during clinical attacks; this may also occur during remission, and in approximately 50% of clinically latent cases.[7]

*Variegate porphyria*

The enzyme primarily affected in variegate porphyria is PROTO oxidase,[17] although the activity of ferrochelatase may also be reduced.[1] As a result, there is overproduction of protoporphyrin and, to a lesser extent, of coproporphyrin, both of which are excreted in excess in the faeces. The increase in faecal porphyrin excretion is greatest during clinical attacks and may be normal in symptom-free relatives with the genetic trait.[19] Overproduction of the

porphyrin precursors ALA and PBG also occurs in variegate porphyria, again varying in accordance with the clinical activity of the
disease.[19]

*Control of hepatic haem biosynthesis*

It is now generally accepted that regulation of hepatic haem biosynthesis is vested in the end-product, haem. Feedback by haem, which
regulates the available activity of the first enzyme, ALA synthase,
occurs by more than one mechanism.[20,21] At the post-translational
level, haem blocks the translocation of pro-ALA synthase into the
mitochondrion.[22] The molecular weights of ALA synthases in the
mitochondrion (59.5 kDa (erythroid), 64.6 kDa (hepatic)) are
smaller than those of cytosolic pro-ALA synthases (64.6 kDa (erythroid), 70.6 kDa (hepatic)).[23] The action of haem on mRNA is to
decrease its stability, and therefore its half-life, thus minimising
protein synthesis.[24]

Most studies to date have concentrated upon hepatic haem synthesis. The erythroid bone marrow is the major haem-forming tissue
in the body, producing 85% of the daily haem requirement. Haem
synthesis in erythroid cells differs from that in hepatocytes: it is
linked to tissue differentiation, and the half-life of the same end-
product is different. Haem complexed with globin is preserved in
circulating red blood cells for approximately 120 days, whereas
haem produced in liver for cytochromes (particularly P450) and
enzymes (eg catalase) is subject to much more rapid turnover,
measurable in hours. Regulation of haem in liver is exquisitely
sensitive to fluctuations in intracellular haem levels because it
needs to respond rapidly to the requirements for synthesis, whereas
a more leisurely response is adequate for haem synthesis in the bone
marrow.

The need for regulation of haem biosynthesis in these two tissues is as different as the ways in which such regulation may be
achieved.[25] Haem in hepatocytes exercises negative feedback on
ALA synthase, but its activity in erythroblasts may be increased by
intracellular haem.[26] This fundamental difference is exemplified by
the two different tissue-specific enzymes and two different cDNAs
for human liver: 'housekeeping' ALA synthase (ALA.S) and erythroid ALA synthase (eALA.S).[27,28] The gene for the hepatic enzyme
lies on chromosome 3,[29] and that for eALA.S on the X chromosome.[30] In accord with the differing control of the two enzymes,
iron-responsive elements (IRE) have been identified on mRNA for
eALA.S. These IREs are probably functional, implying that the
IRE and IRE-binding protein system are involved in the control of
haem biosynthesis during erythroid differentiation.[23,31] It has been

173

suggested that haem regulates its own synthesis by controlling the acquisition of iron from transferrin, rather than by exerting any direct effect on enzyme activity.[32] It is thus clear that haem plays a central role in cell growth and differentiation.[33]

## Preamble to the 1985 and 1990 biochemical studies in Chester

A previously unrecognised form of acute porphyria has been identified in a large family in Chester. Patients presented with attacks of neurovisceral dysfunction, and none has experienced cutaneous photosensitivity. Fifteen years after the pioneering work of Bekerus with this porphyria kindred in the mid-1960s (Chapter 5), blood, urine and faecal samples began to arrive at the porphyria laboratory in the University Department of Medicine, headed by Abraham Goldberg, at the Western Infirmary, Glasgow. Bekerus had noticed that the porphyrin excretion products in samples from the family did not closely match the pattern expected in either acute intermittent or variegate porphyria (Chapter 5). The samples from Youngs and Qadiri's index case (1.6.5.3) were typical of acute intermittent porphyria, but those from the daughter (1.1.6) of one of the brothers of the paternal grandmother of 1.6.5.3 showed the typical excretion pattern of variegate porphyria. Further studies in the family revealed that the excretion pattern among family members varied between these two, with some showing an intermediate pattern.

To clarify this situation, we studied the activities of the haem biosynthesis enzymes and the porphyrin excretion pattern in members of this family compared with those in patients with acute intermittent porphyria and with variegate porphyria. This was published in the *Lancet* in 1985,[34] and is reproduced below by kind permission of the publishers.

During the course of their genetic study in 1990 (Chapter 13), Norton et al[35,36] performed biochemical tests on 73 members of the Chester family, 28 of whom had not previously been tested. Eight new cases of porphyria were discovered, and the porphyria status of two previously tested members was altered. These findings have been incorporated into the family tree (see endpapers). It has not been possible to update the 1985 *Lancet* article by combining the 1990 results because the latter study did not include measurement of leukocyte PROTO oxidase. This enzyme is very unstable and, for the 1985 study, family members had to travel 250 miles to Glasgow.

# Part 2: Chester porphyria: biochemical studies of a new form of acute porphyria*

*KEL McColl, GG Thompson, MR Moore, A Goldberg, SE Church, MR Qadiri and GR Youngs*

## Subjects and methods

### Subjects

*Chester family*. Eighteen members of the Chester family (10 women, 8 men, aged between 20 and 54 years) who were found on initial screening to have either increased excretion of haem precursors (16 subjects) or a normal excretion profile but reduced activity of erythrocyte PBG deaminase (2 subjects) were studied in detail. They were all members of the third and fourth generations of offspring from a marriage in 1888. One patient was having an acute neurovisceral attack when studied. Another patient had a history of acute attacks but was in remission when studied.

*Acute intermittent porphyria*. Thirteen women and six men diagnosed as having acute intermittent porphyria were examined. The diagnosis was based on increased urinary excretion of ALA and PBG, normal faecal porphyrin excretion, and reduced erythrocyte PBG deaminase activity. They were from 14 unrelated families and all aged between 20 and 55 years. At the time of examination seven were experiencing clinical attack, 11 were in remission and one was clinically latent, having never experienced any symptoms of acute porphyria.

*Variegate porphyria patients*. Seventeen unrelated patients diagnosed as having variegate porphyria on the basis of increased faecal porphyrin excretion, consisting predominantly of protoporphyrin, and normal erythrocyte protoporphyrin concentration were examined. Sixteen were women and all were aged between 20 and 55 years. Two were experiencing an attack of neurovisceral dysfunction when examined, 13 had a history of either cutaneous photosensitivity or neurovisceral attacks, but were symptom-free at the time of examination, and two had never experienced any symptoms related to the porphyria.

*Control subjects*. Twenty healthy women and 10 healthy men aged between 20 and 55 years were also studied.

### Laboratory analysis

*Porphyrin and precursor estimations*. Porphyrins and their precursors ALA and PBG were measured in excreta and erythrocytes

*Reprinted, with kind permission of the publishers, from an article in *Lancet*.[24]

Minor editorial changes have been made in accordance with the Royal College of Physicians' house style. References, Tables and Figures have been renumbered consecutively through the chapter.

with the methods described by Moore.[37] Urinary porphyrins were fractionated by means of normal-phase high-performance liquid chromatography.[38]

*Activities of enzymes of haem biosynthesis.* The activities of the enzymes of haem biosynthesis were measured in peripheral blood cells from 50 ml venous blood. The cytosolic enzymes ALA dehydratase, PBG deaminase and uroporphyrinogen decarboxylase were measured in erythrocytes, and the mitochondrial enzymes ALA synthase, coproporphyrinogen oxidase and ferrochelatase in leukocytes.[39] PROTO oxidase was measured in leukocytes with an adaptation of the method of Brenner and Bloomer;[40] the oxidation of PROTO produced by sodium amalgam reduction was measured spectrofluorometrically. It was not possible to measure each of the enzymes in all subjects studied.

*Statistical analysis.* The activities of the enzymes of haem biosynthesis in the different groups were compared by means of the Student *t*-test. The association between the activity of PBG deaminase and the porphyrin excretion pattern was assessed with the Spearman rank correlation.

## Results

*Overproduction of porphyrins and their precursors*

The excretion of porphyrins and precursors and erythrocyte protoporphyrin concentration in each of the groups studied are shown in Table 2.

*Acute intermittent porphyria.* The predominant abnormality in acute intermittent porphyria was increased urinary excretion of PBG; in those in clinical attack it was increased by a mean of 16 times the upper limit of normal and by a mean of 12 times in those who were latent or in clinical remission. The urinary excretion of ALA was also increased but to a lesser extent. Faecal porphyrin excretion was normal except for a very slight increase in coproporphyrin in two of the patients in attack, and a similar increase in protoporphyrin in one patient in remission.

*Variegate porphyria.* The predominant abnormality in variegate porphyria was increased faecal excretion of protoporphyrin; in the two patients in clinical attack it was increased by five times and 12 times the normal upper limit, and by a mean of six times in the clinically inactive cases. Faecal coproporphyrin was also increased, but to a lesser extent. Urinary excretion of PBG was increased in both patients in clinical attack at three times and four times the

**Table 2.** Urinary and faecal excretion of porphyrins and precursors, and erythrocyte protoporphyrin concentration in the different forms of porphyria.

| Subjects | Clinical status | No. | Urinary | | | | Faecal | | Erthrocyte protopor-phyrin§ |
| | | | ALA* | PBG* | Uropor-phyrin† | Coropor-phyrin‡ | Copropor-phyrin‡ | Protopor-phyrin‡ | |
|---|---|---|---|---|---|---|---|---|---|
| Chester family | Attack | 1 | 95 | 295 | 96 | 499 | 59 | 200 | 895 |
| | Remission or latent | 17 | 45 (1–167) | 68 (1–197) | 65 (0–280) | 168 (3.1119) | 126 (18–797) | 457 (37–3057) | 620 (360–900) |
| Variegate porphyria | Attack | 2 | 89 (82 + 96) | 52 (49 + 56) | 134 (95 + 173) | 807 (660 + 954) | 638 (452 + 824) | 1639 (953 + 2325) | 880 (640 + 1005) |
| | Remission or latent | 15 | 44 (1–123) | 29 (1–63) | 72 (8–141) | 420 (44–978) | 466 (66–1400) | 1119 (355–2536) | 860 (468–1085) |
| Acute intermittent porphyria | Attack | 7 | 141 (50–214) | 266 (43–430) | 1057 (284–2043) | 241 (123–399) | 63 (40–96) | 147 (129–168) | 790 (502–991) |
| | Remission or latent | 12 | 113 (9–266) | 197 (5–410) | 171 (4–697) | 130 (42–219) | 64 (38–74) | 189 (7–330) | 803 (498–943) |
| Normal range | | | 0–44 | 0–16 | 0–49 | 0–430 | 0–90 | 0–200 | 300–1100 |

Values given as means with range in parenthesis

* µg/24 hour
† nmol/24 hour
‡ nmol/g dry weitht
§ nmol/l cells

ALA= delta-aminolaevulinic acid
PBG = porphobilinogen

normal upper limit and also in six of the 15 clinically inactive cases by a mean of two times. The eight patients with increased PBG excretion also excreted excess ALA, though to a lesser extent.

*Chester family*. In the Chester family, the excretion pattern varied between subjects. Four of the 18 subjects had normal excretion of porphyrins and precursors. The patient in clinical attack had an excretion pattern typical of acute intermittent porphyria, with a urinary PBG excretion of 18 times the normal upper limit, a less notable increase in ALA, and normal faecal porphyrin excretion. Four of the symptom-free patients also had an excretion pattern typical of acute intermittent porphyria, with the mean increase in urinary PBG 10 times (range 8–12) the upper limit of normal, and normal faecal porphyrin excretion. Four of the symptom-free patients had increased faecal porphyrin excretion, which was predominantly protoporphyrin, with normal urinary excretion of porphyrin precursors; the mean increase in faecal protoporphyrin in these four patients was 2.1 times (range 1.8–2.6) the upper limit of

177

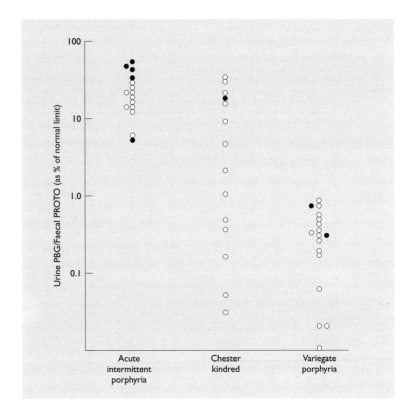

**Fig 4.** Excretion patterns in the different groups of patients studied. The pattern is expressed as a ratio of the urinary porphobilinogen (PBG) excretion (% normal upper limit) over the faecal protoporphyrin excretion (% normal upper limit).

● = clinical attack;
○ = latent or in clinical remission;
PROTO = protoporphyrinogen.

normal. The other five symptom-free patients showed both increased urinary PBG and faecal protoporphyrin excretion; the mean increase in urinary PBG was eight times (range 2–10) the normal upper limit, and faecal protoporphyrin was five times (range 1.3–15) the upper limit. Erythrocyte protoporphyrin was normal in each of these subjects. The ratio of the degree of increased urinary PBG excretion over the degree of increased faecal protoporphyrin excretion for each subject showed clearly the separation between the patients with acute intermittent porphyria, who had ratios varying from 5 to 47, and the variegate porphyria patients, with ratios varying from 0.01 to 0.85 (Fig 4). In the Chester family the ratios varied from 0.03 to 22, and it was possible to classify members into three groups: those with ratios similar to acute intermittent porphyria; those with ratios similar to variegate porphyria; and those with intermediate ratios which fell between the ranges of these two porphyrias. The subjects with these three different porphyrin excretion patterns are shown in a family tree (Fig 5). Acute porphyria was identified in offspring from six of the 10 children from the marriage in 1888. In our studies of the third and fourth generations, the three different excretion patterns appeared to be distributed randomly.

178

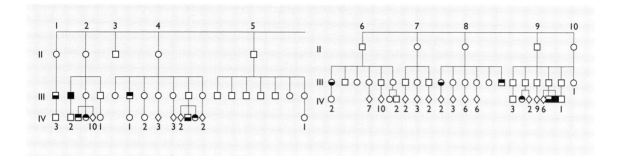

## Activities of the enzymes of haem biosynthesis

The activities of ALA synthase, PBG deaminase and PROTO oxidase in the three study groups are shown in Fig 6. None of the other enzymes studied differed significantly from control values.

*Acute intermittent porphyria.* ALA synthase was increased in each of the subjects with acute intermittent porphyria, with a mean value 10 times that of the controls. The mean PBG deaminase activity was reduced to 54% of the control value. The activities of the other

Fig 5. Family tree of the Chester family showing the relationship of the patients with the different excretion patterns:

□ = males;
○ = females;
◇ = males and females;
◨,◖ = acute intermittent porphyria;
◼,◕ = variegate porphyria;
■ = intermediate.

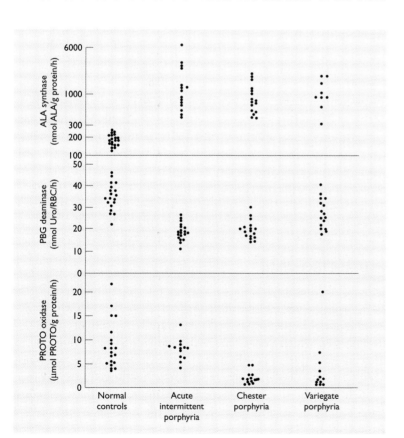

Fig 6. Activities of the enzymes in haem biosynthesis in peripheral blood cells of the three groups of patients studied and in normal controls:
ALA = delta-aminolaevulinic acid;
PBG = porphobilinogen;
PROTO = protoporphyrinogen;
RBC = red blood cells;
Uro = uroporphyrinogen.

enzymes of haem biosynthesis, including PROTO oxidase and ferrochelatase, were similar to control values.

*Variegate porphyria.* ALA synthase was increased in each subject with variegate porphyria with a mean value of seven times that of the controls. The mean PROTO oxidase activity was reduced to 29% of the control value. PBG deaminase was also significantly reduced, with a mean value of 80% of control ($p < 0.005$). Ferrochelatase activity was reduced to a mean of 64% of the control value but, because of the wide range, this difference was not statistically significant.

*Chester kindred.* ALA synthase was increased in each subject with a mean of six times that of the controls. PBG deaminase activity was reduced to a mean value of 58% of the control value. The PBG deaminase was also significantly reduced when compared with that in patients with variegate porphyria ($p < 0.005$) and was similar to that in the patients with acute intermittent porphyria. The mean PROTO oxidase activity was reduced to 23% of the control, similar to that in variegate porphyria. Ferrochelatase activity was reduced to 67% of the control value but, as before, this was not statistically significant.

*Relation of enzyme activities and excretion patterns in the Chester family*

Those members of the Chester family with the lower values for PBG deaminase tended to have an excretion pattern similar to acute intermittent porphyria, and those with the higher values a pattern similar to variegate porphyria, but this was not statistically significant. There was no evidence of any relation between PROTO oxidase activity and the porphyrin excretion pattern.

## Part 3: Discussion

The porphyria we describe does not conform with any of the recognised types of acute porphyria. Biochemically, it produces an excretion pattern which varies in affected individuals from that typical of acute intermittent porphyria to that of variegate porphyria, with some patients showing an intermediate pattern. There are not enough sequential data on individual subjects to know whether these excretion patterns may be seen in the same subject on different occasions. The activities of the enzymes of haem biosynthesis in the Chester family are also different from any previously described porphyria. As in all the acute porphyrias, ALA synthase activity increases considerably in response to the inherited enzymatic block in haem synthesis. However, the Chester family are unusual in that they show reduced activity of both PBG deaminase and PROTO oxidase, the former being reduced to a similar extent to that seen in acute intermittent porphyria and the latter to a similar extent to that in variegate porphyria. The leukocyte PROTO activity in our patients with variegate porphyria is 29% of the control value, which is less than the 50% activity previously reported.[18,41] The explanation for this is not clear but may be related to differences in the white-cell lines studied.

Clinically, the Chester family presented with attacks of neuro-visceral dysfunction common to all the acute porphyrias, and no members experienced cutaneous photosensitivity which may occur in variegate porphyria and hereditary coproporphyria.

There have been a few reports of different forms of porphyria within a family where more than one enzyme is deficient, and Chester porphyria belongs to this group of 'concurrent porphyrias'.[42–48] Watson et al[42,43] reported two cases of cutaneous hepatic porphyria (porphyria cutanea tarda) in a family in which five members had well documented variegate porphyria. Another family has been described in which the father had cutaneous hepatic porphyria, and one daughter was found to have erythropoietic porphyria.[44] Day et al[45] described 25 patients with dual porphyria. These patients belonged to families with well documented variegate porphyria, and were found to have the porphyrin excretion pattern of cutaneous hepatic porphyria superimposed on that of variegate porphyria. In the variegate porphyria families studied by Day, 25% of the porphyria subjects showed this dual pattern, but none was found to have the biochemical pattern of cutaneous hepatic porphyria on its own. Unfortunately, Day was unable to study the activities of the enzymes of haem biosynthesis in his patients with dual porphyria.*

In the Chester family, despite the fact that some patients showed an excretion pattern typical of acute intermittent porphyria and others that of variegate porphyria, the two subgroups did not differ significantly with respect to the activities of the enzymes of haem biosynthesis. All the Chester porphyrics studied had reduced activities of both PBG deaminase and PROTO oxidase, indicating that they probably represent a single genotype with varying phenotype, as expressed in their excretion pattern. The dual enzyme deficiency could produce the different excretion patterns. As shown by patients with acute intermittent porphyria, a 50% reduction in PBG

*The numerous permutations are graphically summarised in Fig 2, from the recent publication by Doss.[48]

deaminase activity may result in overproduction of porphyrin precursors in some patients but not in others.[7] Thus, in some of the
Chester porphyria patients, the reduced PBG deaminase activity
may be the rate-limiting step.

The genetic explanation for the concurrent inheritance of two
different defects within the haem biosynthetic pathway is unclear.
Our observation of reduced PBG deaminase activity in our non-
Chester variegate porphyria patients may be relevant. Meissner
et al[49] found a similar reduction in PBG deaminase activity in variegate porphyria patients in South Africa, though Mustajoki found
normal activity in his Finnish patients.[19] It is possible that the
Chester family represents a variant of variegate porphyria in which
PBG deaminase activity is sufficiently reduced to alter the excretion
pattern.

The dual enzyme defect cannot be explained by proposing that
the Chester family represents double heterozygotes, each having co-
inherited the acute intermittent porphyria and variegate porphyria
genes. If this were the case, these disease loci would be very closely
linked since the two diseases have consistently segregated together
throughout the family. We know, however, that the loci are not jux-
taposed: the locus for PBG deaminase is sited on chromosome 11q[50]
while that for PROTO oxidase is on chromosome 1.[51,52]

Although our studies of the activities of the enzymes of haem
biosynthesis explain the unusual excretion pattern to some extent,
further studies are required of the molecular basis of the enzyme
defects. Such studies of the reduced PBG deaminase activity in acute
intermittent porphyria have shown evidence of genetic heterogeneity, with four mutant classes having a different ratio of catalytic
activity to immunoreactive enzyme protein.[53] Similar studies of
the molecular basis of the reduced PBG deaminase in this Chester
family, and comparison with that of the non-Chester variegate
porphyria patients and patients with acute intermittent porphyria,
may clarify the relation between these different forms of porphyria.
Final clarification should be possible when DNA probes for PBG
deaminase and PROTO oxidase become available.

It has been assumed previously that each type of porphyria is distinct and due to a single enzyme deficiency. However, in addition
to the reduced PROTO oxidase activity in variegate porphyria,
reduced activity of PBG deaminase, uroporphyrinogen decarboxylase or ferrochelatase has also been reported. The name 'porphyria variegata' was first coined by Dean and Barnes[54] because of
the varying clinical manifestations of the disorder. It now appears
that the name is an equally appropriate description of the varying
biochemical picture.

# References

1 Moore MR, McColl KEL, Rimington C, Goldberg A. *Disorders of porphyrin metabolism*. New York: Plenum Press, 1986.

2 Mercer-Smith JA, Mauzerall DC. Photochemistry of porphyrins: a model for the origin of photosynthesis. *Photochemistry and Photobiology* 1984; **39**: 397–405.

3 Rimington C. A reinvestigation of turacin, the copper porphyrin pigment of certain birds belonging to the Musophagidae. *Proceedings of the Royal Society of London, Series B* 1939: **127**: 106–20.

4 With TK. Porphyrins in egg shells. *Biochemical Journal* 1973; **137**: 597–8.

5 Beukeveld GJJ, Wolthers BG, Nordmann Y, Deybach JC, *et al.* A retrospective study of a patient with homozygous form of acute intermittent porphyria. *Journal of Inherited Metabolic Disease* 1990; **13**: 673–83.

6 Hift RJ, Meissner PN, Todd G, Kirby P, *et al.* Homozygous variegate porphyria: an evolving clinical syndrome. *Postgraduate Medical Journal* 1993; **69**: 781–6.

7 McColl KEL, Moore MR, Thompson GG, Goldberg A. Screening for latent acute intermittent porphyria: the value of measuring both leucocyte δ-aminolaevulinic acid synthase and erythrocyte uroporphyrinogen-1-synthase activities. *Journal of Medical Genetics* 1982; **19**: 271–6.

8 Andersson C, Lithner F. Hypertension and renal disease in patients with acute intermittent porphyria. *Journal of Internal Medicine* 1994; **236**: 169–75.

9 Andersson C (ed). *Acute intermittent porphyria in northern Sweden. A population-based study*. Umeå University Medical Dissertations, New Series No. 497. Umeå and Arjeplog, Sweden: University of Umeå and Primary Health Care Centre, Arjeplog, 1997.

10 Macalpine I, Hunter R. The 'insanity' of King George III: a classic case of porphyria. *British Medical Journal* 1966; **1**: 65–71.

11 Macalpine I, Hunter R, Rimington C. Porphyria in the Royal Houses of Stuart, Hanover and Prussia. A follow-up study of George III's illness. *British Medical Journal* 1968; **1**: 7–18.

12 Loftus LS, Arnold WN. Vincent van Gogh's illness: acute intermittent porphyria? *British Medical Journal* 1991; **303**: 1589–91.

13 Dean G. *The porphyrias – a story of inheritance and environment*. London: Pitman Medical, 1963.

14 Whatley SD, Roberts AG, Elder GH. De-novo mutation and sporadic presentation of acute intermittent porphyria. *Lancet* 1995; **346**: 1007–8.

15 Stine OC, Smith KD. The estimation of selection coefficients in Afrikaners: Huntington disease, porphyria variegata, and lipoid proteinosis. *American Journal of Human Genetics* 1990; **46**: 452–8.

16 Meyer UA, Strand LJ, Doss M, Rees AC, Marver HS. Intermittent acute porphyria – demonstration of a genetic defect in porphobilinogen metabolism. *New England Journal of Medicine* 1972; **286**: 1277–82.

17 Brenner DA, Bloomer JR. The enzymatic defect in variegate porphyria: studies with human cultured skin fibroblasts. *New England Journal of Medicine* 1980; **302**: 765–9.

18 Viljoen DJ, Cummins R, Alexopoulos J, Kramer S. Protoporphyrinogen oxidase and ferrochelatase in porphyria variegata. *European Journal of Clinical Investigation* 1983; **13**: 283–7.

19 Mustajoki P. Variegate porphyria. Twelve years' experience in Finland. *Quarterly Journal of Medicine* NS 1980; **194**: 191–203.

20 May BK, Bawden MJ. Control of heme biosynthesis in animals. *Seminars in Hematology* 1989; **26**: 150–6.

21 Andrew TL, Riley PG, Dailey HA. Regulation of heme biosynthesis in higher animals. In: Dailey HA (ed). *Biosynthesis of heme and chlorophylls*. New York: McGraw-Hill, 1990:163–200.

22 Ades IZ, Harpe KG. Biogenesis of mitochondrial proteins. Identification of the mature and precursor forms of the subunit of delta-aminolevulinate synthase from embryonic chick liver. *Journal of Biological Chemistry* 1981; **256**: 9329–33.

23 Cox TC, Bawden MJ, Martin A, May BK. Human erythroid 5-aminolevulinate synthase: promoter analysis and identification of an iron-responsive element in the mRNA. *The EMBO Journal* 1991; **10**: 1891–902.

24 Hamilton JW, Bement WJ, Sinclair PR, Sinclair JF, *et al.* Heme regulates hepatic 5-aminolevulinate synthase mRNA expression by decreasing mRNA half-life and not by altering its rate of transcription. *Archives of Biochemistry and Biophysics* 1991; **289**: 387–92.

25 Abraham NG. Molecular regulation – biological role of heme in hematopoiesis. *Blood Reviews* 1991; **5**: 19–28.

26 Granick JL, Sassa S. Hemin control of heme biosynthesis in mouse Friend virus-transformed erythroleukemic cells in culture. *Journal of Biological Chemistry* 1978; **253**: 5402–6.

27 Bishop DF, Henderson AS, Astrin KH. Human delta-aminolevulinate synthase: assignment of the housekeeping gene to 3p21 and the erythroid-specific gene to the X chromosome. *Genomics* 1990; **7**: 207–14.

28 Watanabe N, Hayashi N, Kikuchi G. Delta-aminolevulinate synthase isozymes in the liver and erythroid cells of chicken. *Biochemical and Biophysical Research Communications* 1983; **113**: 377–83.

29 Sutherland GR, Baker E, Callen DF, Hyland VJ, *et al.* 5-Aminolaevulinate synthase is at 3p21 and thus not the primary defect in X-linked sideroblastic anaemia. *American Journal of Human Genetics* 1988; **43**: 331–5.

30 Astrin KH, Bishop DF. Assignment of human erythroid ALA synthase to the X-chromosome. *Human Gene Mapping 10 Conference Book* 1989: 113–4 (abstract 2329).

31 Dandekar T, Stripecke R, Gray NK, Goossen B, *et al.* Identification of a novel iron responsive element in murine and human erythroid-aminolaevulinic acid synthase mRNA. *The EMBO Journal* 1991; **10**: 1903–9.

32 Ponka P, Schulman HM. Regulation of haem synthesis in erythroid cells: hemin inhibits transferrin iron utilization but not protoporphyrin synthesis. *Blood* 1985; **65**: 850–7.

33 Sassa S. Heme stimulation of cellular growth and differentiation. *Seminars in Hematology* 1988; **25**: 312–20.

34 McColl KEL, Thompson GG, Moore MR, Goldberg A, *et al.* Chester porphyria: biochemical studies of a new form of acute porphyria. *Lancet* 1985; **ii**: 796–9.

35 Norton B, Lanyon WG, Moore MR, Porteous M, *et al.* Evidence for involvement of a second genetic locus on chromosome 11q in porphyrin metabolism. *Human Genetics* 1993; **91**: 576–8.

36 Norton B. A genetic study of Chester porphyria. MD Thesis, University of Liverpool, 1993.

37 Moore MR. *Laboratory investigation of disturbances of porphyrin metabolism*. Association of Clinical Pathologists, Broadsheet 109. London: British Medical Association, 1983.

38 Seubert A, Seubert S. High-performance liquid chromatographic analysis of porphyrins and their isomers with radial compression columns. *Analytical Biochemistry* 1982; **124**: 303–7.

39 Moore MR, Thompson GG, Goldberg A, Ippen H, *et al.* The biosynthesis of haem in congenital (erythropoietic) porphyria. *International Journal of Biochemistry* 1978; **9**: 933–8.

40 Brenner DA, Bloomer JR. A fluorometric assay for measurement of protoporphyrinogen oxidase activity in mammalian tissue. *Clinica Chimica Acta* 1980; **100**: 259–66.

41 Deybach J Ch, de Verneuil H, Nordmann Y. The inherited enzymatic defect in porphyria variegata. *Human Genetics* 1981; **58**: 425–8.

42 Watson CJ, Cardinal RA, Bossenmaier I, Petryka ZJ. Porphyria variegata and porphyria cutanea tarda in siblings: chemical and genetic aspects. *Proceedings of the National Academy of Sciences of the USA* 1975; **72**: 5126–9.

43 Watson CJ, Cardinal RA, Bossenmaier I, Petryka ZJ. Porphyria variegata and porphyria cutanea tarda in siblings: chemical and genetic aspects (addendum). *Proceedings of the National Academy of Sciences of the USA* 1976; **73**: 1323.

44 Levine J, Johnson WT, Tschudy DP. The coexistence of two types of porphyria in one family. *Archives of Dermatology* 1978; **114**: 613–4.

45 Day RS, Eales L, Meissner D. Coexistent variegate porphyria and porphyria cutanea tarda. *New England Journal of Medicine* 1982; **307**: 36–41.

46 Doss MO. New form of dual porphyria: co-existent acute intermittent porphyria and porphyria cutanea tarda. *European Journal of Clinical Investigation* 1989; **19**: 20–5.

47 Nordmann Y, Amram D, Deybach JC, Phung LN, Lesbros D. Coexistent hereditary coproporphyria and congenital erythropoietic porphyria (Günther disease). *Journal of Inherited Metabolic Disease* 1990; **13**: 687–91.

48 Freesemann AG, Hofweber K, Doss MO. Coexistence of deficiencies of uroporphyrinogen III synthase and decarboxylase in a patient with congenital erythopoietic porphyria and in his family. *European Journal of Clinical Chemistry and Clinical Biochemistry* 1997; **35**: 35–9.

49 Meissner PN, Sturrock ED, Moore MR, Disler PB, Maeder DL. Protoporphyrinogen oxidase, porphobilinogen deaminase and uroporphyrinogen decarboxylase in variegate porphyria. *Biochemical Society Transactions* 1985; **13**: 203–4.

50 Meisler MH, Wanner L, Kao FT, Jones C. Localization of the uroporphyrinogen 1 synthase locus to human chromosome region 11q13→qter and interconversion of enzyme isomers. *Cytogenetics and Cell Genetics* 1981; **31**: 124–8.

51 Roberts AG, Whatley SD, Daniels J, Holmans P, *et al*. Partial characterization and assignment of the gene for protoporphyrinogen oxidase and variegate porphyria to human chromosome 1q23. *Human Molecular Genetics* 1995; **4**: 2387–90.

52 Taketani S, Inazawa J, Abe T, Furukawa T, *et al*. The human protoporphyrinogen oxidase gene (PPOX): organization and location to chromosome 1. *Genomics* 1995; **29**: 698–703.

53 Mustajoki P, Desnick RJ. Genetic heterogeneity in acute intermittent porphyria: characterisation and frequency of porphobilinogen deaminase mutations in Finland. *British Medical Journal* 1985; **291**: 505–9.

54 Dean G, Barnes HD. Porphyria in Sweden and South Africa. *South African Medical Journal* 1959; **33**: 246–53.

# Chapter 13

# The genetics of the Chester porphyria

BERNARD NORTON AND MICHAEL CONNOR

As with any genetic study, the first steps in the investigation into the genetics of Chester porphyria were to:

- draw up a reliable family tree;
- establish the pattern of inheritance; and
- obtain suitable samples for analysis from as many family members as possible.

Thanks to the hard work of many others, notably Giles Youngs, a large family tree had already been constructed (see endpapers), and the pattern of inheritance is clearly autosomal dominant – that is, affected individuals have a 50% chance of passing on the affected gene to any of their children. Suitable samples for genetic analysis included samples of blood for DNA extraction, together with urine and faeces for confirmation of Chester porphyria status.

## Sampling the Chester porphyria kindred

The next task was to recruit to our study as many family members as possible, both affected and unaffected, together with the spouses and adult offspring of the affected members. Three factors quickly became apparent that would help in these endeavours:

- the high fecundity in the kindred;
- the fact that the majority of the family had remained local to the Chester area; and,
- most importantly, the kind cooperation which was virtually universal throughout the family.

Laboratory analysis for porphyria status was carried out by Professor Michael Moore at the Gardiner Institute, Western Infirmary, Glasgow. Analysis of the blood, urine and faecal samples was sufficient in the vast majority of cases to establish individuals as either affected or unaffected. Disease status was assigned on the basis of clinical and family history, together with quantification of porphyrins and their precursors in urine, faecal porphyrins and red cell porphobilinogen deaminase levels. In addition, 28 previously untested family members were tested, eight of whom were identified as new cases.

## DNA analysis

Human DNA exists in complementary pairs of long strands of only four nucleotide bases: adenine, thymine, guanine and cytosine. Restriction enzymes, of which there are several hundred each with its own specific recognition site, occur naturally in many bacteria and cut double-stranded DNA only at specific sequences. A restriction digest is made by incubating DNA with a restriction enzyme until each recognition site in the DNA has been cut. Typically, this can produce over a million smaller fragments of various sizes from a genomic DNA sample. Each restriction fragment length polymorphism represents the presence or absence of a particular site, and is a normal inherited difference between DNA of healthy people. Gene probes are small strands of radiolabelled DNA which will bind to their complementary strand within a mixture of DNA fragments.

DNA restriction analysis consists of first digesting the DNA with a restriction enzyme and separating the resultant fragments according to size by gel electrophoresis (Fig 1). The DNA fragments are then transferred to a filter by Southern blotting. Exposure to the radiolabelled probe produces a specific banding pattern on an autoradiograph (X-ray photograph). The presence of a DNA polymorphism will result in a different banding pattern; if a combination of several polymorphisms is examined simultaneously, the result is specific to an individual: the so-called 'genetic fingerprint'.

### Genetic polymorphisms

These genetic polymorphisms can be exploited to determine the chromosomal location of human genes. All human chromosomes contain an abundance of polymorphisms, and highly detailed maps have been constructed showing the exact position on each chromosome of commonly occurring genetic polymorphisms. Linkage (or closeness together on the chromosome) is the occurrence of a polymorphism adjacent to the disease gene in question, and hence their co-inheritance. By studying DNA samples obtained from a large cohort of related individuals with a genetic disorder, it is

188

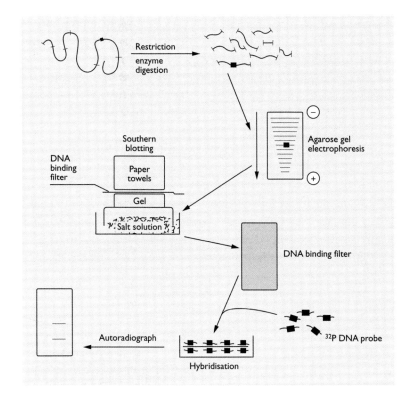

**Fig 1.** Restriction analysis of DNA.

possible to test a battery of polymorphisms to see whether any are co-inherited. If linkage between the particular gene and any one of these markers can be established, the gene will reside at the same chromosomal location. The tighter the linkage, the closer the marker will be to the gene in question.

At least 150 different polymorphic markers are required to cover the entire human genome. Closely related genes often arise from duplication and subsequent divergent evolution of a common ancestral gene. Although the resultant genes may eventually be separated on to different chromosomes, several examples are known where they have remained in fairly close proximity on the same chromosome (eg the beta-globin gene family).

## The Chester porphyria gene

*The search begins*

The starting point for the genetic search in the Chester kindred was therefore the established chromosomal loci known to harbour the genes of other forms of acute porphyria:

- porphobilinogen deaminase (PBGD): chromosome 11q for acute intermittent porphyria;[1,2]

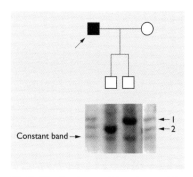

**Fig 2.** *Taq* I polymorphism detected by PEFD126.3:

□ = males;

○ = female;

■ = porphyria gene inherited.

- alpha-1-antitrypsin: chromosome 14q for variegate porphyria;[3]
- markers from chromosome 9q for hereditary coproporphyria: coproporphyrinogen oxidase.[4]

The investigation of chromosomal regions 9q, 14q and 11q was carried out by testing for linkage with either restriction fragment length DNA polymorphisms or variable numbers of tandem repeat polymorphisms (minisatellites) from those areas.

In contrast to the restriction fragment length or site polymorphisms, the polymorphic nature of minisatellites is secondary to an inherited variation in genetic length between two constant restriction sites. The DNA polymorphisms were selected on the basis of:

- proximity to the area under scrutiny;
- high heterozygosity rate of the relevant alleles in the general population (heterozygosity being a prerequisite for phase-known meioses from affected individuals); and
- availability of the corresponding gene probes.

*Chromosome 14q.* This chromosome was investigated using a biochemical marker, alpha-1-antitrypsin, phenotyping. The different protease inhibitor (PI) phenotypes were distinguished by alteration in electrophoretic mobility using isoclectric focusing in polyacrylamide gels.[5]

*Chromosome 9.* There was no evidence for linkage with the chromosome 9 markers, as can be seen from the example given in Fig 2. The male subject (arrowed) is positive and has two unaffected sons. The bands represent the markers (one from each chromosome) for each of the four individuals. He and his wife have two bands, and are therefore heterozygous with respect to the marker (ie each of them has produced two different fragments). The two unaffected sons, however, are opposite homozygotes. If the Chester porphyria were linked to this particular marker, we would expect one of the sons to be positive. Discordant segregation in this and other branches of the family thus excludes this region of the genome. Similar results were obtained with chromosome 14.

## Location of the Chester porphyria gene to chromosome 11q

In contrast, tight linkage was observed with an *Msp* I polymorphism using probe PICJ52.208M2 from the long arm of chromosome 11. This linkage is demonstrated in Fig 3. The index female case deceased (arrowed) was affected. She had married twice: from her first marriage, she had one unaffected and three affected children and, from her second, three affected and two unaffected children (bands represent the restriction fragment phenotype for each person).

190

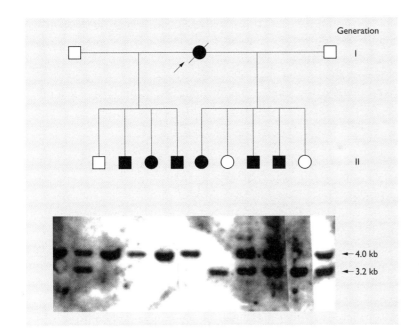

**Fig 3.** *Msp* I polymorphism detected by PICJ52.208M2:
□ = males;
○ = females;
■ = porphyria gene inherited.

Although the index case is deceased, we can infer that she is an obligatory heterozygote for this marker as she has opposite homozygous children. The first husband is homozygous for the larger restriction fragment (top band), and contributes this allele to each of his four children. The unaffected child has received the smaller fragment, whereas the three affected children have all received the larger fragment from their affected mother (in addition to the Chester porphyria gene).

Her second husband is a heterozygote (two bands present), and only the first two and the fifth children are informative meioses – that is, it can be said with certainty which of the two marker alleles was received from which parent. The first child, who has inherited the Chester porphyria gene from her mother, is homozygous for the larger fragment, and hence must have inherited the mother's larger fragment at meiosis. The second and fifth children are negative for the Chester porphyria gene; they are both homozygous for the smaller fragment, and hence must have received the mother's smaller fragment.

The odds of this marker linking with the disease in this way by chance is $1/2^7$ or 128 to 1: that is, the chance of the larger restriction fragment allele being inherited together with the Chester porphyria gene and of the smaller allele passing with the normal gene.

In genetic studies, it is customary to refer to the logarithm of the odds (LOD) score, which in this particular branch of the family alone is just over 2. The rest of the family was tested with this

191

marker, and it was found to track with the disease throughout the family with only one recombinant observed. The recombinant was a young girl who was clearly affected with Chester porphyria, but who – alone among the other affected members of the kindred – had inherited the smaller marker allele from her affected mother rather than the larger allele.

*Recombination*

Recombination, which occurs at meiosis, is the normal exchange of genetic material between chromosome pairs. Unless genes are located extremely closely together, recombination will result in a percentage of otherwise linked genes being separated. The tighter the linkage between two genes – or, in our case, gene and marker – the less frequently will the recombination events separating them occur. Consequently, the percentage of recombinants or recombination fraction becomes smaller – approaching zero. The further apart the two genes are on a chromosome, the more the recombination events will occur, rising to a maximum of 50%, as would be expected by chance alone for genes on different chromosomes.

By convention, a maximum LOD score value above 3 (corresponding to an odds ratio of 1,000:1) is accepted as establishing the presence of linkage at the corresponding recombination fraction.[6] The PICJ52.208M2 marker gave a maximum LOD score of 5.25 at a recombination fraction of 0.07 (7%), thus locating the Chester porphyria gene to the long arm of chromosome 11.

## Chester porphyria is distinct from acute intermittent porphyria

The locus for acute intermittent porphyria, cPBGD, also lies in 11q, so it was necessary to look for linkage with the cPBGD locus to determine whether or not the Chester porphyria locus is at a separate position. Ten informative meioses were observed with a polymorphism at the cPBGD locus, and a minimum of four recombinants identified with Chester porphyria – which is compatible with independent assortment. The maximum LOD score was negative at −0.14 at a recombination fraction of 0.40 (40%). These results confirmed that Chester porphyria is distinct from acute intermittent porphyria.

Other markers from this region then had to be examined to pinpoint more accurately the exact location of the Chester porphyria gene on chromosome 11. The position of each of the markers on chromosome 11, their distance apart, and the degree of linkage exhibited by each to the Chester porphyria gene all contribute to the assignment of the Chester porphyria locus. This task required a large amount of data analysis. Multipoint linkage analysis was performed using the LINKMAP program.[7] The location scores generated were converted into LOD scores, and plotted graphically against distance in centimorgans (cM) (approximately 1 million base-pairs) to construct a linkage map and determine likelihood calculations for the position of the disease locus. In essence, the linkage data for each marker is programmed into the computer, which gives relative likelihoods for the Chester porphyria gene locus as the proposed locus is moved along a fixed set of points in this region. The peak LOD score represents the most likely position for the gene to be located.

The multipoint analysis was performed using the 11q markers CRI-L424, PMCT128.1/0.9, PICJ52.208M2, L7 and cPBGD to determine the position of the Chester porphyria locus. The marker order and distances apart were derived from the consensus map of 11q (Human Gene Mapping 11[8,9]). LOD scores were computed over a distance of 30 cM, covering points coincident with each marker at equidistant intervals between markers and at distances of up to 10 cM outside the marker group. A maximum LOD score of 7.33 was obtained at a distance of less than 1 cM proximal to D11S351 (locus of the PICJ52.208M2 marker). These findings confirmed the linkage between Chester porphyria and D11S351 observed on two-point analysis. LOD scores of greater than 3 were seen extending over a distance of 8 cM around this locus.

The localisation of the Chester porphyria gene to 11q can be determined more precisely by further linkage analysis using both two-point and multilocus mapping with other polymorphic markers from this region.

## Benefits of localising the Chester porphyria gene

One immediate benefit of localising the Chester porphyria gene is the use of linked DNA markers as a diagnostic test in the identification of family members at risk of inheriting the disease. This would be particularly important in the detection of pre-symptomatic cases and where the biochemical findings are equivocal. Ideally, it should be possible to isolate flanking markers, one mapping either side of the disease locus, to leave only double recombinants as a rare source of error in diagnosis.

The use of linked markers to track genes in suitably informative families is now an established method of diagnosis. This localisation also allows identification of potential candidate genes which can be screened with mutational analysis strategies. Once the gene is identified, this will both allow improved genetic counselling and also open prospects for gene therapy, in addition to providing further insight into the biochemical pathway of porphyrin metabolism.

## References

1 Meisler MH, Wanner L, Kao FT, Jones C. Localization of the uroporphyrinogen 1 synthase locus to human chromosome region 11q13→qter and interconversion of enzyme isomers. *Cytogenetics and Cell Genetics* 1981; **31**: 124–8.

2 Wang AL, Arredondo-Vega FX, Giampietro PF, Smith M, *et al*. Regional gene assignment of human porphobilinogen deaminase and esterase A4 on chromosome 11q23→11qter. *Proceedings of the National Academy of Sciences of the USA* 1981; **78**: 5734–8.

3 Bissbort S, Hitzeroth HW, du Wentzel DP, Van den Berg CW, *et al*. Linkage between the variegate porphyria (VP) and the alpha-1-antitrypsin (PI) genes on human chromosome 14. *Human Genetics* 1988; **79**: 289–90.

4 Grandchamp B, Weil D, Nordmann Y, Van Cong N, *et al*. Assignment of the human coproporphyrinogen oxidase to chromosome 9. *Human Genetics* 1983; **64**: 180–3.

5 Allen RC, Harlcy RΛ, Talamo RC. A new method for determination of alpha-1-antitrypsin phenotypes using isoelectric focusing on polyacrylamide gel slabs. *American Journal of Clinical Pathology* 1974; **62**: 732–9.

6 Morton NE. Sequential tests for the detection of linkage. *American Journal of Human Genetics* 1955; **7**: 277–318.

7 Lathrop GM, Lalouel JM, Julier C, Ott J. Strategies for multilocus linkage analysis in humans. *Proceedings of the National Academy of Sciences of the USA* 1984; **81**: 3443–6.

8 Junien C, van Heyningen V. Report of the committee on the genetic constitution of chromosome 11: chromosome 11. *Cytogenetics and Cell Genetics* 1991; **58**: 459–54.

9 Julier C, Nakamura Y, Lathrop M, O'Connell P, *et al*. A detailed genetic map of the long arm of chromosome 11. *Genomics* 1990; **7**: 335–45.

*Chapter 14*

# Perspective

GILES YOUNGS

The endeavours of the junior doctors Shaper and Bekerus in 1954 and 1963–65, respectively, and latterly my own team, have uncovered the medical misfortunes of a remarkable family suffering from a disease which hoodwinked medical practitioners in Chester for several decades. With hindsight, it is easy to spot the delayed or inaccurate diagnoses leading to inappropriate management over the years. Much of this was obvious to the family, such that one symptomatic member, having lost several of his young cousins, limited his own family to one child. Family members at times had the additional burden of scant sympathy and accusations of hysteria from their medical advisers.

I hope our enquiry has uncovered some influences which mitigate this tale of woe. The clinical aspects of the acute hepatic porphyrias were accurately described only immediately before the second world war by Waldenström, and thereafter by Goldberg, Dean and Eales. Porphyria was thus not in the medical school curriculum of many of the early medical advisers of our family, and the concept of 'continuing medical education' was as yet unborn. The porphyrias are rare diseases and many physicians will not see a case during their career. Above all, our family's experience demonstrates the dangers posed by a rare disease masquerading as a more common ailment – abdominal pain, psychiatric disturbance or neuritis. So diverse are the clinical presentations that porphyria does not fit comfortably into any one specialty, curriculum or textbook; instead we find rather brief mention in textbooks of gastroenterology, haematology, psychiatry and inborn errors of metabolism. There is no national or international clinical porphyria society or journal.

The organisation of medical care in Chester also explains the delay in defining the enigma. It is to be expected that the primary care of the family was divided between different general practices, but for most of this century our city of 80,000 inhabitants and a catchment area of 220,000 people had hospitals on four separate sites – all with radiological departments and three with operating theatres. Care was thus compartmentalised and fragmented. Joint academic activities were rare. Only in 1996 were we amalgamated.

The final mitigating influence was the universal practice of prescribing barbiturates for conditions as diverse as epilepsy, neurosis and psychosis, hypertension, and also for anaesthesia and as an aid to sleep. My wife remembers being prescribed barbiturates for this last purpose in 1965 when she was revising for nursing examinations and found sleep difficult because she was on night duty. In that era, the medical profession was more paternalistic and judgemental; any change for the better since then is more due to change in society than to doctors themselves seeing the light. I wonder which of our current prescribing practices – polypharmacy perhaps? – will be vilified three decades hence.

The demography of the family has fascinated me. Peter Dobson has over 330 offspring to date, and only three of his 38 grandchildren left Chester – both factors of great help for our study. The Malthusian spread of Peter Dobson's genes has thus been local, and the consequences in keeping with the concept that 'genes drive society'. It could have been different: had the family scattered throughout the country, it is unlikely that this story would have been put together – illustrating the concept that in this modern age of social mobility 'society drives genes'. It remains conjectural why such a high proportion of grandchildren carried the porphyria gene – and, of course, all family studies of this sort are subject to the vagaries of genetic paternity. In this respect, members of our Chester kindred are no different from their peers, there being several single-parent families.

It is also conjectural why there is such a high gene penetrance resulting in symptomatic as opposed to latent porphyria in our family compared with other porphyria families. It could be the type of mutation, the level of expression of the other allele, the effect of other loci, or non-genetic factors. One or more of these factors might similarly explain why so often in our family a symptomatic member has a latent parent and vice versa.

The opportunities for repeating a study such as this in the future may be few and far between. The Swedish study by Waldenström, Andersson and Lithner, Dean's South African study, Andrews' Plymouth study, and hopefully our Chester study, may remain as landmarks.

I hope this monograph conveys some of the fascination of the Chester porphyria. It must be this fascination that motivated the pivotal contribution of junior doctors to this study. All but two of the 10 junior doctors and co-authors of this monograph were in one-year posts accredited for general professional – not higher specialist – training. Their main requirement was to pass the MRCP examination, not to do research, yet they alone often provided succour to the family members – a bond which was then broken as they moved on. Shaper in 1954 might not have diagnosed porphyria had he not seen cases as a medical student in South Africa. Bekerus might not have embarked on her study if the nursing sister had not reported the red urine in her patient. But for their intervention, other family members may well have received barbiturates with disastrous consequences.

Many of the family's medical attendants in the early years must have been sorely perplexed at their patients' bizarre symptoms and signs, and stretched to provide plausible diagnoses and death certificates while trying to maintain the dignity of their professional position. So it is that when facing an undiagnosable patient on a ward round I wonder how often I am a victim of the same predicament and am staring at a diagnosis well described in the textbooks.

As a young consultant in 1974, I joined my colleagues for waitress-served lunch in the boardroom at the Chester Royal Infirmary. This privilege was soon swept away, so reducing the opportunity for the interdisciplinary communication so relevant to porphyria, even though we are now all on one site in Chester.

We also have to contend with changing medical practice. As a medical student on Clifford Wilson's renal firm at the London Hospital in 1963, I had to test all my patients' urine samples. Now I rarely see a urine specimen, and so would miss the port wine colour of the porphyric subject. Alan Bennett[1] tells us that King George III's medical adviser, Sir Henry Halford, like Bekerus, benefited from his assistants' observations on the colour of the urine – two of the King's pages argued whether the royal urine was blue or purple. The subsequent film script settled for blue and raised the eyebrows of students of porphyria. Wilfred Arnold[2] advises us to reserve our scorn, arguing (rather improbably, I feel) that the King's constipation, a common feature of porphyric crisis, may have led to increased urinary excretion of indican (indoxyl sulphate) which, by bacterial action, changed to indigo blue.

We now have a porphyria register and information sheets for our family members and colleagues in general and hospital practice. An advice sheet on the management of porphyric crisis is included in the ward protocol book, although happily admissions of family members are rare nowadays – quite why is difficult to say. In our catchment population of nearly a quarter of a million people, we know of only one non-family case of acute hepatic porphyria. We and family members are still frustrated by equivocal biochemical results when trying to decide the porphyria status of an asymptomatic subject, important when questions concerning contraceptive and other drug advice arise. The cut-off between normal and low levels of porphobilinogen deaminase is not distinct. We have been grateful for the services of the porphyria laboratory in Glasgow, now sadly closed, and currently of that in Cardiff. Let us hope a reliable genetic test is not too far away, and that in the future gene therapy for porphyria will be feasible.

We are left with a final conundrum – the use of the eponymous possessive. Dr Ronald McClure wrote of his patient having 'Dobson's complaint', but many family members were afflicted so should it be 'Dobsons' complaint'? Carothers[3] and Anderson[4] tell us that the use of the eponymous possessive in the medical press is confusing and inconsistent, but the trend is to drop the possessive. Neither author mentions eponyms derived from families as opposed to individuals. Porphyria provides another family example – van Rooyen's skin, the epithet coined by members of the branch of the South African kindred with variegate porphyria.[5] If we were to drop the possessive, should the title of this monograph be Dobson or Dobsons complaint? Doubtless my publisher has strong views on the matter, and I await the edict.

We have told a story about a fascinating malady affecting a remarkable family. Many of them have experienced bad times, but without their cooperation this study would not have been possible.

## References

1 Bennett A. *The Madness of King George III*. London: Faber & Faber, 1992.

2 Arnold WN. King George III's urine and indigo blue. *Lancet* 1996; **347**: 1811–3.

3 Carothers AD. Continuing confusion over the eponymous possessive (letter). *British Medical Journal* 1995; **311**: 1508.

4 Anderson JB. The language of eponyms. *Journal of the Royal College of Physicians of London* 1996; **30** :174–7.

5 Dean G. *The porphyrias – a story of inheritance and environment*. London: Pitman, 1963.

# Glossary

## Family notation

Our description of the family in the *British Medical Journal*[1] labelled each generation with the Roman numerals I–IV, and the members of each generation in Arabic numerals:

- 1–10 for the children of Peter Dobson and Sarah Pay,
- 1–40 for their grandchildren, and
- 1–109 for their great-grandchildren.

In his MD thesis,[2] Norton numbered only the 67 great-grandchildren who had porphyria-positive parents. On receiving Bekerus' documents in 1989, which were written in 1965 (Chapter 5), we were interested to find that she had used a similar system. However, this notation has the drawbacks, first, that any new member, either by birth or error of omission, necessitates altering the notation of all subsequent members of that generation and, secondly, it does not give information of parentage. The new notation that we have developed labels each individual in the order of birth amongst siblings, and repeats the notation of the parent and grandparent. Thus:

| | |
|---|---|
| Peter Dobson (married 1888) | |
| Eldest child | 1.1 |
| Eldest child of eldest child | 1.1.1 |
| Second child of eldest child | 1.1.2 |

*Example*: Subjects 1.5.2.1, 1.5.5.7 and 1.8.2.1 are all great-grandchildren of Peter and Sarah Dobson. The first two are cousins, being grandchildren of Peter and Sarah's fifth child, the third is a second cousin, being a grandchild of their eighth child.

The new notation omits members who died before reaching adult life, so that there are 38 grandchildren and 106 great-grandchildren rather than 40 and 109 in the two generations given in the *British Medical Journal*.

## Terms used in this book

*Obligatory carrier*: a member by birth of the Chester kindred deemed to carry the porphyria gene because one or more of his or her off-spring have porphyria. This assumes the genetic paternity or maternity shown on the family tree.

*Symptomatic, overt or manifest porphyria*: a person with porphyria who has experienced typical neurovisceral symptoms.

*Latent porphyria*: a person with genotypic porphyria who has never had neurovisceral symptoms. This includes persons with hypertension or renal failure who are otherwise asymptomatic.

## References

1 Qadiri MR, Church SE, McColl KEL, Moore MR, Youngs GR. Chester porphyria: a clinical study of a new form of acute porphyria. *British Medical Journal* 1986; **292**: 455–9.
2 Norton B. *A genetic study of the Chester porphyria*. MD thesis, University of Liverpool, 1993.